2—
2/23

Is Heart Surgery Necessary?

Is Heart Surgery Necessary?

WHAT YOUR DOCTOR WON'T TELL YOU

JULIAN WHITAKER, M.D.

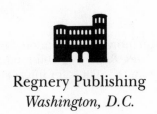

Regnery Publishing
Washington, D.C.

Library of Congress Cataloging-in-Publication Data

Whitaker, Julian M.
    Is heart surgery necessary? : what your doctor won't tell you / Julian Whitaker.
        p.   cm.
    Includes bibliographical references and index.
    ISBN 0-89526-473-0
    1. Coronary heart disease—Popular works. 2. Coronary heart disease—Treatment. 3. Surgery, Unnecessary. I. Title.
RC685.C6W47 1965
616.1'206—dc20   95-10587
                                            CIP

Published in the United States by
Regnery Publishing, Inc.
An Eagle Publishing Company
422 First Street, SE, Suite 300
Washington, DC 20003

Distributed to the trade by
National Book Network
4720-A Boston Way
Lanham, MD 20706

Printed on acid-free paper.
Manufactured in the United States of America

10 9 8 7 6 5 4 3 2 1

Books are available in quantity for promotional or premium use. Write to Director of Special Sales, Regnery Publishing, Inc., 422 First Street, SE, Suite 300, Washington, DC 20003, for information on discounts and terms or call (202) 546-5005.

To my wife, Jutta; my children,
Jay, Conrad, Luisa, and Max;
and my parents,
Dr. William and Lesee Whitaker.

CONTENTS

Acknowledgments   ix
Introduction: Why I Gave Up Being a Surgeon
                To Become a Healer   xi

PART I: AVOIDING THE HEART SURGERY TRAP

1 Scared Into Surgery   3
2 What Your Doctor Won't Tell You About
        Bypass Surgery   13
3 Should I Have a Bypass?   29
4 Angiograms: Slippery Slope to Surgery   43
5 Angioplasty: Two Steps Backward   53
6 Women and Heart Surgery   63
7 Money and Medicine   69

PART II: THE REAL CAUSES OF HEART DISEASE

8   What Is Heart Disease?   77
9   Free Radicals: Where Heart Disease Begins   83
10 The Cholesterol Controversy   93
11 The Truth About Fats   101
12 What About Blood Pressure?   111

PART III: THE WHITAKER WELLNESS PROGRAM

13 Getting Well With the Four Pillars of Therapy   119

The First Pillar: Food for the Heart

14 The Best Medicine   131
15 The Right Fats   139

16 The Healthy Heart Diet Plan   145

17 Recipes From the Whitaker Wellness Institute   161

The Second Pillar: Nutritional Supplements

18 Starving Amidst Plenty   175

19 Antioxidants: The Big Three   181

20 State of the Art Supplements   189

21 Miracle Mineral   201

22 Back From the Dead   205

23 Healing Waters   215

24 What About Your Prescription Drugs?   219

The Third Pillar: Progressive Exercise

25 The Easy Way to a Healthy Heart   229

The Fourth Pillar: EDTA Chelation Therapy

26 The Cure That Could Replace Surgery   247

27 The Healing Mind   257

28 Health and Healing   263

Appendix: Where to Find What You Need   269

Notes   273

Index   279

ACKNOWLEDGMENTS

I have great admiration for the true visionaries of the world, those who grasp an idea before its time and work to see it realized, often in the face of public criticism and ridicule. The fortunate ones are able to experience the fruits of their labors, while others persevere without reward.

In this category I would place the doctors and researchers on the VACS and CASS teams who did the initial research, revealing the truth about bypass surgery, and others, such as Eugene Braunwald and Henry McIntosh, who saw the truth for what it was. Thomas Graboys, Philip Podrid, Bernard Lown... these are a rare breed of cardiologists who have heeded the scientific literature demonstrating the risks of the invasive approach to heart disease.

I want to acknowledge the entire "alternative medicine" community of researchers, practitioners, and patients who want more than what conventional medicine has to offer. They are visionaries. In my office, we don't refer to our approach as "alternative medicine." We call it "good medicine."

I would like to thank the following people at Regnery Publishing who have contributed a great deal of time, energy, and heart in making this book a reality: Editors Richard Vigilante, Stephen Weeks, and Jamila Abdelghani; marketing and promotion manager Jennifer Reist; and editorial assistant David Dortman.

I would also like to acknowledge my research assistant, Peggy Dace, of the Whitaker Wellness Institute, who has labored on this project from the beginning.

Why I Gave Up Being a Surgeon To Become a Healer

Heart disease is the number one killer in this country. Half of all Americans who die this year will die from heart disease and related cardiovascular illnesses. The causes of these ailments are known, and there are proven treatments that can prevent or reverse the condition. These treatments are painless and noninvasive. But the disease continues to kill more than a million people every year.

Almost half the people who will die of heart disease do not even know they have it. Annually some 400,000 people die suddenly, with no previous signs of angina. When someone dies of heart disease, it is listed as a "natural cause." Yet dying of clogged arteries is no more natural than being run over by a truck.

The medical profession is doing something about heart disease, but it is doing the wrong thing. Instead of promoting exercise, nutrition, and lifestyle changes that are inexpensive and that have been proven effective, doctors are constantly recommending and performing heart surgery that is dangerous and expensive. Every year, 400,000 patients with heart disease have bypass surgery: their chests are ripped open, and a vein or artery from their leg is grafted onto their diseased heart. Does this procedure make them better? Not often. Does it cure the disease? Not at all. Then why do they submit to it?

Because they are afraid. They have been frightened into surgery by doctors who tell them, "You have a ticking time bomb in your chest; you'll be lucky if you make it to Christmas." The doctors often don't tell their patients that bypass surgery is dangerous, that it doesn't cure heart disease, and that it might kill them.

It is often difficult to recognize that the simplest solution tends to be the most effective one. With a proper diet and healthy lifestyle you can prevent heart disease, stay out of the hospital, and live a long and productive life.

You can avoid the heart surgery trap. I have been using my diet, exercise, and supplement program for fifteen years on thousands of patients and have found it to be extraordinarily beneficial for almost every one of them. So, what's the big secret? Something that a lot of doctors won't tell you: You can control your own health and make yourself better.

I come from a medical family. My father is a prominent surgeon in Atlanta, Georgia, one of the most skillful and compassionate surgeons I've ever known. He's been honored on numerous occasions, including having a Chair of Surgery founded in his name at the hospital where he served for many years as chief of surgery. My older brother is a radiologist in

Atlanta and was president of his county medical association. He is also highly respected in his field.

I have known since I was ten years old that I wanted to be a doctor. I got my undergraduate degree from Dartmouth College, where I found I had an aptitude for science that enabled me to excel in courses some other premeds found difficult. I entered the medical school at Emory University in the fall of 1966.

In medical school you have to digest so much material you don't have time to question what you're being taught. We all believed what we were learning was relevant and up-to-date.

I was no different from most medical students. I worked hard. I learned what I was told to learn. I graduated from Emory University Medical School thirteenth in a class of about ninety students.

I entered a medical-surgical internship at Grady Memorial Hospital in Atlanta, the busiest hospital under Emory's teaching wing. My work load increased. After completing my internship I entered an orthopedic surgery residency at the University of California in San Francisco.

It was there that I began to have misgivings about my profession and my place in it. Surgeons get their greatest degree of personal satisfaction from the drama of surgery, rather than working with patients. I began to believe that something was dreadfully wrong with the medical profession's focus on surgery, drugs, and other risky procedures. I felt that we had reached a point in scientific advancement where we needed not little changes around the edges, but a complete paradigm shift in the way medicine is practiced and the way health is perceived. With all this weighing heavily on my mind, I dropped out of the four-year surgical program to reevaluate my goals.

I went to southern California and began working in the Kaiser Hospital emergency room. There I encountered a thirty-four-year-old woman who had sprained her ankle. I noted that, aside from her ankle, she absolutely radiated health. Her skin glowed, her eyes sparkled, her hair looked alive. I had never seen a patient in her state of health. Then it dawned on me that a physician rarely sees—and certainly does not interact with—truly healthy people.

My first healthy patient started to tell me about herself. She was a Shaklee representative. She took a lot of vitamins and minerals, exercised regularly, and followed a healthy diet. I was intrigued. She steered me to Dr. Wilbur Currier, a physician in Pasadena who had given up a career in ear, nose, and throat surgery to specialize in nutrition and preventive medicine. I visited Dr. Currier and, shortly thereafter, started working in his office.

Dr. Currier was one of the first physicians to support a little-known inventor by the name of Nathan Pritikin, who had written about low-fat nutrition as therapy for heart disease, diabetes, and high blood pressure. Dr. Currier loaned me one of Pritikin's early monologues on diabetes, and I remember being astounded by what I had not been taught in medical school.

Mr. Pritikin referred to numerous articles dating back to the 1920s and 1930s which clearly demonstrated that a high carbohydrate diet helped treat diabetes—that it could eliminate the need for insulin in some patients and certainly improve the condition for all of them. I had never been taught to use nutrition as a therapeutic tool. Virtually no doctors are today. So I was amazed at how clearly the research and the medical literature supported the idea.

I visited Pritikin at his center, which was then in Santa Barbara, and joined his staff in 1976. In the eight months I was there, the direction of my medical career changed irrevocably. For the first time in my entire medical training, I actually understood what it meant for patients to get well.

By this time in my career, I'd admitted and discharged hundreds of patients, and although many of them had improved, without exception, none had actually gotten well. Yet, in just one month at Pritikin's center, I saw people with diabetic conditions throw away their insulin. I saw patients lower their blood pressure enough to get off medication. I saw angina pain simply disappear.

At that point I knew I would devote the rest of my career not manipulating patients' bodies to bring about short-term relief from symptoms but teaching patients how to make themselves well.

THE WHITAKER WELLNESS INSTITUTE

In 1979, I started the Whitaker Wellness Institute, a residential program for patients with heart disease, diabetes, high blood pressure, and obesity. My patients were housed in a hotel rather than a hospital. After a complete medical evaluation, they were put on a very low fat diet, with vitamins and minerals and other food supplements, and started on an exercise regimen.

In the fifteen years since, I have treated thousands of heart patients and have seen almost all of them reverse or prevent further heart disease and live happier and healthier lives. I have counseled many of them to avoid the heart surgery trap, and they have successfully treated themselves with safe and effective methods of diet, exercise, and nutrition.

I've also incorporated other nonsurgical therapies, such as EDTA chelation therapy and more sophisticated supplements, into my practice as I have learned about them. As I witnessed the efficacy of simple, holistic medical practices and the success of noninvasive, nonsurgical techniques, I also watched the medical profession go in the opposite direction, toward more and more surgery that was more and more dangerous, traumatic, expensive, and unnecessary.

In recent years there has been an explosion of surgical procedures for all kinds of ailments, but particularly for heart disease. For someone who has seen the power of diet, lifestyle change, and noninvasive therapy, the negative effect of today's expensive and debilitating approaches to heart disease is profoundly disturbing.

There are times, of course, when invasive therapies are appropriate and necessary. But I believe that many or most heart surgeries are unnecessary and harmful to the patient. I know that my treatment methods are less harmful and more effective. Cardiovascular disease is not difficult to treat, and the most powerful tools available are simple and inexpensive.

THE WELLNESS PROGRAM

My Wellness Program is not a single corrective procedure in which the doctor repairs the patient as a mechanic might fix his car. In my program, the doctor guides and teaches. The patient learns the treatment and heals himself.

I refuse to accept the quality of health care that most Americans settle for. Even though I come from a family of doctors and have great respect for the profession, I have always felt that there has to be a better way. In that spirit, this book has three purposes:

- To alert you to recognizing the dangerous nature of heart surgery.

- To help you decide if surgery is right for you.

- To show you how to take charge of your own healing and achieve lasting wellness.

By reading this book and following my recommendations, you can live a long and healthy life, and you can avoid the heart surgery trap.

PART ONE

Avoiding The Heart Surgery Trap

CHAPTER ONE

Scared Into Surgery

Millions of Americans have been pushed into dangerous heart surgery that's wrong for them. You can say no.

John had enjoyed good health for a long time when, at age sixty-three, he began having chest pains. Then, with almost no warning, he had a heart attack. He was rushed to the hospital, where his doctors discovered he had a serious blockage in a crucial artery bringing blood to his heart. That blockage had caused the heart attack. His doctors told him that unless it was dealt with immediately, he could have another, fatal, attack at any time. The only solution, they said, was multiple bypass surgery. With no apparent alternatives, John consented.

Within a few hours he was being prepped for surgery. As with every bypass patient, John was shaved of all body hair from the chin down to protect him from infection. A bypass procedure actually consists of two operations at once, one incision on your chest and another even longer incision down your leg.

John's operation followed normal procedure. Once a patient is under anesthesia, the chest is cut open along the breastbone, which is then split down the middle with an electric saw. The rib cage is retracted with an exceptionally strong instrument, called a rib spreader, exposing the heart and lungs to full view. Once a patient's chest is opened, the pericardial sac, which covers the heart, is cut and peeled away from the heart muscle.

Next the doctors stopped John's heart so it could be operated on. The heart pumps blood to the lungs, where it receives oxygen; the oxygenated blood returns to the heart and is pumped throughout the body. If the brain is deprived of oxygen for only four minutes, it begins to sustain permanent damage and the patient is at risk of death. So, John was hooked up to the heart-lung machine, a device without which bypass surgery would be impossible.

For the duration of the operation the heart-lung machine takes over the function of oxygenating and pumping the blood. Large tubes are inserted into the patient's venous system, which normally carries blood back to the heart, and the arterial system, which carries blood away from the heart. With the tubes in place a flick of the switch shunts all this blood through the machine. The patient's heart is then stopped by an infusion of potassium.

Bypass surgery is used to compensate for blockages in one of the several arteries carrying blood from the aorta into the heart. A harvested vein is needed as a "bypass" to carry blood from the aorta to which it is grafted to a place on the blocked artery "downstream" from the blockage. In John's case the surgeons created three separate bypasses to ensure adequate blood flow and to guard against the consequences of blockages developing in one or two of the grafts themselves. The grafts came from the patient. While the heart surgeon was

BYPASS SURGERY

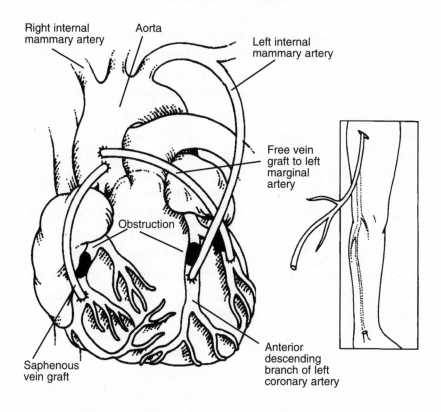

Right internal mammary artery

Aorta

Left internal mammary artery

Free vein graft to left marginal artery

Obstruction

Saphenous vein graft

Anterior descending branch of left coronary artery

opening John's chest, another surgeon harvested a nonessential vein from his leg to make the actual bypasses.

The operation must be done rapidly. Once on the heart-lung machine the patient literally begins to die. The machine starts inflicting damage to the brain and to all other organs the minute it is turned on. A patient who remains on the machine too long—and ninety minutes can be too long—is risking death. Patients who survive an extended period on the machine may experience tragic complications, including total memory loss, cognitive dysfunction, and emotional disorder.

Even a short stay on the machine under the most skillful hands will cause some brain damage.

With the graft successfully in place the retractors are removed from John's rib cage and his chest bone is rejoined with heavy stainless steel wire. The skin incisions are closed, and John is transferred to an ICU with tubes in nearly every orifice. As he awakens he is confused, experiences personality changes and memory loss, and has difficulty concentrating. Other patients have hallucinations, seizures, or strokes. Up to 5 percent may sustain long-lasting or permanent cerebral damage. About 4 percent die on the table or within a few weeks of the procedure. (This is called *perioperative death,* occurring either during surgery or within thirty days.)

John was lucky. He had no unusually serious complications, and the surgery appeared to be a success. He felt well for about five years. Then the nightmare started all over again. The chest pains were back and John's doctor urged him to have another operation. Once again his doctor told him he would surely die without it.

But John did not want the surgery; he'd had enough. So, he came to see me.

THERAPY, NOT SURGERY

When I saw John, he could not even walk across the parking lot to my office without experiencing shooting pains in his chest. John had come because he knew I opposed surgery in most cases and prescribed a nonsurgical medical course of treatment for most of my patients. Yet after seeing John even I thought that surgery was probably indicated, and I told him so. But he would have none of it.

So, I started him on an "aggressive-conservative" treatment program for heart disease. The treatment was "conservative" in that we would avoid surgery unless and until it was clearly necessary, and it was "aggressive" in that John would start a medical regimen, including drug therapy, exercise, and nutrition, far more intensive than most doctors prescribe for their heart patients.

For drug therapy I kept John on his regular heart medication, calcium channel blockers and nitroglycerin, drugs designed primarily to forestall another heart attack while John got well.

Then I started him on a four-point plan designed to return him to good health.

We began with a very low fat diet and a carefully planned, moderate, progressive exercise program. I had to push John to keep him active, since at first he could hardly walk without chest pains. Many doctors believe exercise aggravates heart problems. But lack of exercise can be far more dangerous. The answer for serious heart patients is careful, supervised exercise.

The third part of the program was a vitamin and nutritional supplement regimen: John began taking water-soluble B-complex vitamins as well as an antioxidant supplement regimen of vitamin C, vitamin E, and beta carotene. Antioxidants defend the artery walls from "free radicals," which come from oxidized fat molecules and are linked to arterial plaque buildup. But John needed more: I also put him on three nutrients that specifically strengthen the heart muscle: L-carnitine, coenzyme Q10, and magnesium.

The fourth part of the plan was EDTA chelation therapy, which targets heart and vascular disease. EDTA, which is given intravenously, seeks out minerals inside the body, especially heavy metals such as mercury, lead, and cadmium, and attaches to the minerals, making them water soluble so they can be easily excreted. EDTA chelation therapy cleanses the body of problematic mineral deposits that harden the arteries and contribute to heart disease. John thrived on it.

Full Recovery

John improved almost immediately. His cholesterol level dropped from 284 to 147 in one month. His pain subsided just as quickly, and he found he could walk farther and farther without angina.

John first came to me on August 3, 1990. In March 1991 he climbed to the top of the Statue of Liberty with no pain and no shortness of breath. Three months later, he climbed to the top of the Torre del Mangia in Siena, Italy, and only had to catch his breath twice. He has never regretted saying no to surgery.

Clearly John's cardiologists and surgeons were wrong in their "surgery or else" prediction. John did not need bypass surgery to avoid a heart attack. He did not need surgery to regain his health or alleviate his pain. And contrary to their repeated denials when John asked the doctors if there were any alternative therapies, there was another way out.

Standard Operating Procedure

John's story is not an uncommon one. Some 400,000 bypass operations are performed in America every year. The average cost of such an operation today is about $40,000. For most categories of patients (there are important exceptions), the survival rate of those who refuse surgery is higher than the survival rate of those who go for the operation, even though many who refuse never undertake the kind of regimen I prescribed for John. Even the *Journal of the American Medical Association* has said that 44 percent of bypass surgeries are of questionable necessity.

In reality the number of unnecessary heart surgeries is far higher than that. In fact, most operations are worse than "unnecessary," since they are always dangerous and frequently counterproductive. Even the two leading surgical alternatives to bypass surgery—angioplasty and atherectomy—billed with partial accuracy as being cheaper and safer than bypass, can be dangerous and ineffective, damaging the arteries, making new blockages more likely, and giving the unwitting patient a false sense of security, thus making a second, and perhaps fatal, heart attack more likely.

The scientific evidence damning most (though not all) heart surgery is overwhelming. The right, noninvasive medical therapies are, on average, successful and, on average, atherectomy, angioplasty, and bypass surgery are not. Despite the mountains of evidence, cardiologists and surgeons continue to recommend risky operations promiscuously.

SCARED INTO SURGERY

Many of today's heart doctors use scare tactics as standard operating procedure. In some cases, it seems as if the more the patient resists the doctor's prescription, the more frightening the doctor becomes. All too many patients go into hospitals to be "evaluated" for chest pains, only to find that the evaluation has become an angioplasty or bypass before they can even leave the hospital to get a second opinion.

I've had hundreds of frantic phone calls from heart patients and their relatives "trapped" in hospitals facing just this problem. Their concerns are always the same:

- How can I just walk out?

- What if my doctor is right; do I really have time to wait for a second opinion?

- My insurance will pay for bypass, but it won't cover alternative procedures.

- They tell me I don't have much time, and bypass seems so quick and sure compared with the alternatives.

- Is there a doctor in my area who will treat me immediately if I choose not to have surgery?

- Have I waited too long for the alternatives to be effective? Is it really too late, as my doctor suggests?

- My doctor is telling me I'll be dead before Christmas if I don't have a bypass. How can I say no to that?

And worst of all, these questions are put to the patient in a manner more suited to a used car lot than a medical consulting room:

- They want my decision now!

When patients find themselves facing a life-and-death decision in a hospital—the most emotionally charged atmosphere possible—the three crucial factors ruling a decision to have surgery or refuse it are rarely discussed rationally:

1. *What is the real statistical risk this particular patient faces of dying from his particular heart difficulties without surgery? In many, and perhaps most cases cardiologists exaggerate the risk.*

2. *What is the patient's actual risk of death or other serious harm (including new blockages) from the surgery itself and how does that risk compare with the risks of other therapies?*

3. *How suited is this particular patient to alternative nonsurgical therapies?*

Without considering each of these points a patient will not have the information to make this momentous decision. Too often ill-informed patients act out of fear, thinking that a second opinion is a luxury they can ill afford.

That's wrong. The overwhelming majority of patients undergoing bypass surgery can afford to wait and are better off if they do. For them surgery—dangerous and debilitating physically, financially, and psychologically—is no more effective than medical therapy.

NEEDED: A NEW LIFESTYLE

The nonsurgical approach I recommend addresses the causes of heart disease and can substantially reverse it. It is a powerful therapy for angina and will strengthen the heart, lower blood cholesterol and blood pressure, decrease "stickiness" of the blood, and actually reverse blockages in the arteries.

Of course there is no guarantee that the aggressive-conservative nonsurgical approach will prevent heart attacks or reverse blockages in every patient. Neither can the heart surgeon or cardiologist guarantee that you won't die on the table. But the nonsurgical approach to heart disease, including heart medications and lifestyle changes, has been clearly demonstrated to be not only the most powerful treatment available, but in most cases also the safest.

I have found that even patients aware of alternatives to invasive cardiac procedures often don't have the strength or support to seek them out. Changing one's lifestyle is not easy. Taking responsibility for your own health can be a lot harder than just giving in to the man with the knife who promises to solve all your problems while you are asleep on the table. And those who say "no" to bypass will do so in the face of much opposition.

To protect themselves patients need all the facts about the surgical treatments the cardiology establishment is promoting today. Bypass and the other surgical techniques are brilliant technological innovations. And they can be lifesavers. But more often they are abused or overused. The sad fact is that you cannot automatically rely on a heart doctor's recommendation to have surgery. Information is power. Learning the facts about your heart will empower you to make the right decisions, instead of simply appealing to the authority of a man in a white coat.

If you or your loved one are considering heart surgery, you do not have to be a helpless victim. By using this book you can become an informed patient, with the power to make the right choices about your body.

THE RIGHT CHOICE

John made the right choice, and he is now leading a healthy and active life. He's in the best shape ever, without having to undergo another painful, dangerous, and debilitating round of surgery. John's never regretted refusing surgery. He didn't give in to fear. And neither should you.

CHAPTER TWO

What Your Doctor Won't Tell You About Bypass Surgery

Does bypass work?
How dangerous is it?
What are the side effects?

Bypass surgery does not cure or prevent heart disease. At best it is a palliative, easing the severity of the disease without curing it. At worst it can kill you.

A cardiologist in Baltimore recently told a patient: "You have really bad blockages. You need an operation. With an operation, you'll live another fifteen years. Without the operation, don't get any subscriptions. Buy the magazines off the rack."[1]

This kind of fear tactic is used all the time. First the doctor told his patient that he needed the operation; it wasn't presented as an option. Then he promised that the seventy-one-year-old patient would live to be eighty-six with the surgery. Finally, and harshly, he threatened the patient that without the surgery he would not live out a year.

None of this was true. Unfortunately for the cardiologist, he happened to say this in front of a *Washington Post* reporter. Most of what is said in a doctor's office doesn't get reported.

Heart doctors often turn their prognosis into a threat: "If you do not have this operation, you could be dead in six months," or, "You have a ticking time bomb in your chest."

Once you have that image of a ticking time bomb in your chest, even if your doctor then acts responsibly and tells you that your chances of recovery without surgery are good, there is no way you'll be able to think about anything but that ticking time bomb. Would you board a plane if there were a bomb aboard, even if there were only a 5 percent chance of it going off?

There are a whole lot of statistics concerning heart surgery, and I'm going to use a few of them. In evaluating these data, there's an important thing to keep in mind. You are not a statistic. You are a human being with unique needs. You may be one of the minority who actually requires bypass surgery. Or you may be one of the many for whom bypass would be a mistake.

THE HISTORY OF BYPASS

Let's take a look at the history of invasive cardiac procedures. In 1950, surgeons had the idea that tying off the mammary artery, which delivers blood to the chest, would increase blood flow through the coronary arteries and reduce chest pain. They began operating on patients, and the results of this "miracle" surgery were dramatic. Ninety percent of their patients claimed improvement in pain and symptoms. But in most cases the improvement lasted only a few months.

Soon the procedure was being prescribed routinely. Yet it was not until ten years later that it was scientifically tested in a controlled study. Surgical candidates were told they were going to undergo the procedure, and all of them were prepped, anesthetized, and cut open. But though all the patients were led to believe they had had the surgery, only half actually had the mammary artery tied off; the others just had their chests opened and closed.

After the operation all the patients noted diminished pain, but there was no improvement in the ability to exercise in either group. Researchers were dismayed to find that the placebo group received the same benefit as the group who had their arteries tied.

The study effectively ended this procedure, but others followed, each new invasive procedure being hailed as the ultimate solution until it too was disproved.

Then, in the 1960s, medical researchers developed two important technologies. One was the angiogram, an X-ray technique that allows arterial blockage to be pinpointed and evaluated. The other technology was the heart-lung machine, which keeps patients alive while their hearts are stopped for graft placement. These two developments eventually made bypass possible.

While there are some reports of a successful heart bypass operation being performed at Baylor College of Medicine in 1964, it is commonly accepted that the first bypasses were done almost simultaneously by two different surgical teams a few years later. Rene Favaloro and his colleagues at the Cleveland Clinic and Dudley Johnson et al. in Milwaukee both performed successful operations in early 1967. Studies of the procedure began coming out in 1968, and soon the surgery was being practiced at most major cardiac centers.

EFFECTIVENESS OF BYPASS

It was not until the mid-1970s, by which time tens of thousands of operations had been performed, that the first scientifically controlled studies of bypass took place. And when the results finally did start coming in, it became clear that bypass wasn't the miracle cure it was purported to be. Significant among the medical literature are two major long-term studies (and their more recent follow-ups) that have seriously called into question the usefulness of bypass surgery for most patients.

The Veterans Administration Cooperative Study

The first major study of the results of bypass was the publicly funded Veterans Administration Cooperative Study (VACS),[2] the results of which were published in the *New England Journal of Medicine* in 1977.[3] In this trial, 596 males with heart disease were randomly assigned to either a surgical or a medical group. The surgical group of 286 patients got bypass surgery, while the medical group of 310 patients continued with their regular therapy.

At the end of the trial three years later, the difference between the two groups' survival rates was statistically insignificant. The surgical group had a survival rate of 88 percent, and the medical group's survival rate was 87 percent.

Since it had already been proven that patients with left main artery disease had improved survival rates from surgery, the researchers did not include these patients, and the survival rates of both groups listed above reflected the exclusion of left main patients. Instead they focused on the other, lower risk patients.

If bypass is meant to extend the life of low-risk heart patients, then in this respect, it was a failure. Except in the case of left-main patients, the surgery was at best irrelevant. But of the patients who underwent surgery, the perioperative mortality rate was 5.6 percent. That means 16 of the 286 patients died from the surgery, which was about average for that time. (Though mortality rates vary greatly among different hospitals, they have, on average, gotten better. But there is still a significant risk of death for today's patients.)

The VACS report occasioned enormous controversy and criticism from bypass proponents. Their criticism stimulated another controlled trial, again funded with public money.

The Coronary Artery Surgery Study

The Coronary Artery Surgery Study (CASS) began shortly after the VACS results were published. The researchers sought out surgical centers with the highest patient volumes, the lowest death rates, and the most experienced surgeons and cardiologists. The results were shocking.[4]

All of the 780 selected patients had suffered either a heart attack or chest pain from heart disease for at least six months. All had a 75 percent or greater blockage in one, two, or three of the heart's main arteries.

Translation: These were not healthy people; these were patients with very serious heart problems.

Half of the group had surgery, while the other half continued with conservative medical therapy. The surgical group had a perioperative mortality rate of 1.4 percent, which is low for bypass. And 6.4 percent of them had heart attacks during the operation, another low rate for that time. After five years, the two groups were statistically identical. The nonsurgical group had an annual mortality rate of 1.6 percent, while the surgical group had an annual mortality rate of 1.1 percent, but that figure does not include the 1.4 percent perioperative mortality. Once again the difference was statistically insignificant. The annual survival rate for those who refused surgery this time was even better than in the case of the VACS nonsurgical group—more than 98 percent.

CASS researchers concluded: "patients similar to those enrolled in this trial can safely defer bypass surgery until the symptoms worsen to the point that surgical palliation is required."

The term "surgical palliation" means operating to ease pain, not to cure the patient.

CASS: THE FOLLOW-UP TEN YEARS LATER

A ten-year follow-up study on the CASS patients was published in 1990, comparing the death rates of the medical and surgical groups.[5] The numbers were still statistically identical. About 80 percent of both groups were still alive. The researchers again concluded that bypass surgery did not prevent heart attacks or cardiac death.

"It's remarkable that there was no difference in total survivorship of these patients after 10 years," Dr. Lawrence Cohen of Yale University, a coauthor of the study, told the *New York Times*.[6] Why was he so surprised? All previous literature pointed toward the same conclusion. The CASS follow-up did nothing but restate the lesson that should have been learned in the original study: In all but extremely sick patients, bypass surgery does not prolong life.

The VACS and CASS studies are the most comprehensive and reliable studies of bypass results. But the findings of numerous other studies in recent years are, if anything, more discouraging to bypass fans, perhaps because much of the more recent data reflect the results from bypass surgery under average conditions, whereas the operations performed under the CASS experiment were performed under optimum conditions.

In case you're still not convinced, here's a sampling of some of the most recent data concerning bypass surgery.

Another VACS and Its Follow-up

In the eight-year follow-up of another group of Veterans Administration heart patients, 468 patients were randomized into high- and low-risk groups.[7] High-risk patients were those who had three or more diseased vessels and a left ventricle ejection fraction of less than 60 percent. Those with less than three-vessel disease and a left ventricle ejection fraction of more than 60 percent were characterized as low risk.

Among the 181 low-risk patients, cumulative mortality, after eight years of follow-up, was significantly lower in the medically treated patients (16.8 percent) than in the group that had surgery (31.2 percent).

Harvard Gets With the Program

A recent study by Harvard medical professors, which analyzed outcome data on more than 200,000 heart patients, found that invasive surgical techniques often have little effect on long-term survival.[8] The study, which examined nationwide hospital discharge data for Medicare patients who suffered heart attacks, suggested that bypass and other surgeries could be reduced at least 25 percent without increasing mortality.

The study also found that while patients who were treated at top-rated heart centers did tend to have longer survival rates than those who were treated at smaller hospitals, the quality of surgery had little to do with these results. The reason patients survived better at the cardiac centers was due to the noninvasive therapy available at these hospitals, especially during the first twenty-four hours of their treatment.

Much of the data concerning survival rates at different hospitals should be considered in light of this report. Is a hospital's low mortality rate due to the quality of its top heart surgeons, or is it due to the other unsung medical professionals who help the patient fight heart disease himself?

EuroCASS

The European Coronary Artery Surgery Study (EuroCASS) Group came out with a study in 1988 that purported to prove that bypass patients had a much higher survival rate than those treated medically.[9] But when they looked at the same patients years later, they were forced to conclude that "the patients originally assigned to surgical treatment who survived to five years fared worse than those in the medically treated group, and the benefit of early surgical treatment gradually decreased."

EuroCASS also found that patients who underwent surgery had just as many subsequent heart attacks as those who were treated medically. It is important to remember that in all these studies surgery is being compared to standard, nonsurgical medical therapy, not to the advanced techniques in the "aggressive-conservative" regime used by my patients and those of other doctors who follow the "aggressive-conservative" path. It is possible that many of the medically treated patients in these studies could have done much better using some of the techniques I will describe in this book. The point is that Harvard's surgery is no better and maybe worse than Harvard's standard medical therapy for many patients.

Not only does bypass not cure heart disease, it also does not extend longevity in most patients. Does it at least provide the heart with more oxygen? Yes, for a while. But bypass is just a quick fix that often doesn't last long.

A Temporary Fix

Even successful bypass surgery is only a temporary palliative. Dr. Harvey Simon of Harvard Medical School, reviewing the current literature, notes that "after five years, 40 percent of bypass grafts are at least partially blocked, and after 10 years the failure rate is about 75 percent."[10]

This is hardly news. Researchers have known for years that bypass actually promotes heart disease. "There's quite a bit of evidence that disease develops in the grafts and they don't stay open," says Katherine Detre of the Veterans Administration Medical Center in West Haven, Connecticut, who coordinated the 1984 VACS study.

The scientific studies examining reclosure of grafted veins provide damning evidence. A major study published in the *New England Journal of Medicine* concluded that progression of significant heart disease—defined as a loss of 25 percent or more of the lumen (the cavity of a tubular organ)—was more than ten times as frequent in bypassed arteries as in those that were not operated on. The researchers concluded, "These findings support the view that minimally diseased coronary arteries should not be bypassed."[11]

Why does bypass promote heart disease? As we will see more fully in a later chapter, the buildup of "plaque," the material that makes blockages, begins when the cells on the walls of the artery are damaged. Without this damage to the cells, the fatty deposits from which plaque begins have nothing to hold onto. But once the artery walls are damaged, plaque begins building, attracting other materials like calcium and muscle cells that harden the arteries and block the blood flow.

When the doctor sews a vein from your leg onto a coronary artery and connects that to your aorta, he is creating arterial damage. Studies show that the buildup of plaque is most significant in the areas where the surgery has been performed. "Fifty to 90 percent of significant artery stenosis [blockages] proximal to a vein graft become more severe or occlude severely within 5 years of surgery."[12] That is medicalese for saying that most bypass grafts are themselves blocked within five years, and that blockage occurs close to the graft.

The vessel itself is often healthy, but blockages occur near both ends of the graft where the surgeon has allowed heart disease to develop by damaging the tissue of the arteries.

Angina also returns over time. Studies have reported recurrence rates of 20 to 40 percent within three to five years. And after ten years there is no significant difference in angina between surgical and medical groups.

Bypass also gives you a false sense of security. You have been treated surgically by medical professionals who tell you that you're now "good as new." The pain of angina has gone away, at least temporarily—your heart is, for now, getting more oxygen. Under these circumstances it's very easy to slip back into the lifestyle habits (no exercise, fatty diet, smoking) that put you under the knife to begin with.

THE DANGERS OF BYPASS

Bypass is a very dangerous operation. Knowing all about these risks is an important factor in deciding whether you should submit to it. In the case of patients with severe heart disease, sometimes the risks are worth it. But in many prospective bypass patients, the dangers far outweigh any possible benefits.

Side Effects of the Surgery

All surgery is traumatic. But bypass surgery is about the most traumatic form of surgery there is.

If you submit to bypass surgery, there's a 1 to 5 percent chance that you'll suffer a major stroke. If you're over sixty-five, there's a one in three chance that surgery will be followed by a heart attack, coma, stroke, kidney failure, or death.

A joint committee of the American Heart Association and the American College of Cardiology found that 75 percent of patients had neurobehavioral defects after surgery.

A study by the Rand Corporation showed that 24 to 79 percent of patients have declines in cognitive function after bypass.[13]

In one study published in the British medical journal *Lancet*, six patients undergoing bypass were examined by MRI (magnetic resonance imaging).[14] Brain swelling occurred in all six patients within the first hour after surgery.

Dr. John Murkin, an anesthesiologist on the open-heart surgery team at the University of Western Ontario, headed a study that tested such factors as hand-eye coordination, reflexes, and short-term memory of three hundred patients before and after bypass. Half of his patients had lower scores following surgery.

"Their psychological and neurological performance was clearly impaired," Murkin told *Omni* magazine.[15] And his concern was echoed recently by a six-nation study published in 1990, which found that a person after bypass runs a high risk of stroke, severe cases of anxiety and depression, and even hallucinations. This study concluded that bypass was more traumatic than any other surgery. Again it estimated that 50 percent of all patients were affected.

These psychological and neurological side effects are possibly caused by microemboli, tiny particles and gas bubbles that enter the circulation and block the blood flow to the brain, causing a stroke. The microemboli get into the bloodstream through the heart-lung machine, as it pumps carbon dioxide into the blood (to make up for the loss of CO_2 when the blood is cooled to minimize tissue damage to the heart).

Other risks that could cause brain damage include variations in blood pressure, the level of red blood cells maintained during the surgery, and the way the patient is cooled and warmed. All of these could affect the amount of oxygen reaching the brain. And, just like the heart, if the brain does not get oxygen, it starts to die.

Among the other side effects of bypass surgery are pneumonia, hemorrhage, heart attack, cardiac causalgia (intense, burning pain), irregular heartbeat, bursting wounds, and reoperation due to reclosed grafts.

With each repeated procedure, the risks increase geometrically. Reopening the sternum is risky, because the pericardium was left open from the first operation to prevent compression and the risk of hemorrhage. This leaves the heart dangerously exposed. Perioperative mortality of repeat bypass patients can reach as high as 17 percent. Reoperation is also problematic because scar tissue forms after the initial operation, and the best veins have already been harvested from the leg. It also requires longer operating time, because the old grafts must be removed. This means more time on the heart-lung machine, and an increased risk of the side effects associated with it.

Caution: This Procedure Could Kill You

The worst side effect of bypass surgery is, of course, death. While the death rates at specific hospitals can range anywhere from zero to 52 percent, the national average is about 3 to 5 percent. Would you fly on an airline if one out of twenty of their flights crashed?

Deaths on the operating table can occur from a heart attack or stroke. Some patients suffer congestive heart failure because the heart muscle is damaged during the operation and loses its ability to contract. If that happens a transplant becomes the patient's only hope. Many of them die. In other patients the heart does not restart after being taken off the heart-lung machine. The number of patients who die because their hearts cannot be restarted is estimated to be around three thousand per year.

Bypass Causes Heart Attacks

Yet another side effect of bypass is heart disease. Every year some ten thousand people who have had bypass surgery die from heart attacks (that does not include the 5 percent who suffer from heart attacks during the surgery itself). Since the surgery is supposed to prevent a heart attack, these numbers are troubling. There is one possible explanation, and it doesn't bode well for the fans of bypass.

In most of these postoperative heart attacks, the vessels themselves look fine. But the artery and branches beyond the graft (or, in angioplasty, beyond the opened blockage) are constricted.

Doctors at Stanford University Medical Center have shown that these arteries constrict because they are trying to recreate the blood flow they were used to before the operation.[16] While there was blockage upstream from them, the arteries grew accustomed to a very low blood flow. Once that blockage was opened up with angioplasty or bypassed with a graft, the arteries clamped down to recreate the low blood flow. The more significant the previous blockage, the more the downstream arteries constricted. Because the change was radical and immediate, rather than organic and gradual, the vessels reacted in defense of what they perceived to be a change for the worse.

The Stanford researchers have found that these arteries constrict within thirty minutes of surgery and stay constricted, negating the effects of the operation before the patient even comes out of anesthesia.

Cruel and Unnecessary Treatment

How many bypass operations are unnecessary? Nearly half, according to a Rand Corporation study published by the *Journal of the American Medical Association* in 1988.[17]

The researchers studied 386 coronary bypasses performed at three randomly chosen hospitals in three different years. They reported that only 56 percent of the operations were appropriate, under a definition developed by a nine-member panel of doctors to assess whether the benefits outweighed the risks.

By eliminating the unnecessary operations, the report concluded, doctors could cut costs and at the same time improve patient care.

Since the release of that study, the number of bypass surgeries has increased by more than 50 percent. In 1987 there were 230,000 operations. In 1990, 392,000 bypasses were performed.

LAST OPTION

It is now clear that bypass does not cure heart disease and that in most cases the patient can avoid it without ill effect. Bypass should be considered as a last option, rather than a first resort. The scientific data proving the ineffectiveness and overuse of bypass surgery are now overwhelming. Saying that bypass surgery is often unnecessary and always dangerous is about as scientifically sound as predicting that water will boil at 212 degrees Fahrenheit. Yet these data are being continually ignored. That is, despite the preponderance of scientific evidence against them, bypass and other invasive heart surgeries are still being performed at an alarming rate, and the rate is increasing every year.

SHOULD YOU HAVE BYPASS?

So many family members have told me that when their loved ones died during bypass surgery, the doctor, after expressing his sympathy most sincerely, hastened to say that he had done all he could. Perhaps he should have just left the patient alone.

You should consult with at least two doctors when considering heart surgery. But there are also some simple guidelines to help you decide whether you need the operation. In the next chapter I'll tell you what criteria to use in helping to make this important decision—how to find out whether you really do need bypass surgery, or whether you're just another victim caught in the heart surgery trap.

CHAPTER THREE

Should I Have a Bypass?

A few good reasons and many bad reasons for bypass.
How to get a second opinion.

Although bypass is always dangerous and often ineffective, there are some patients who should have it. If your heart disease is serious enough, bypass may be an option—a drastic option, but one that should not be dismissed before weighing all the facts.

There are a few good reasons to have bypass surgery, and many bad ones. The following guidelines can help you decide what to do. But they should be supplemented. You should also read the literature, consult with doctors, talk with your loved ones. Don't make a hasty decision; heart surgery is a matter of life and death.

GOOD REASONS FOR BYPASS

The following situations are good reasons for bypass:

➤ *Significant blockages in the left main coronary artery.*

➤ *An "ejection fraction" (a term I will explain in a moment) of less than 50 percent.*

➤ *Three or more arteries significantly blocked, and decreased left ventricular function.*

➤ *Incapacitating chest pain.*

If you have one or more of the above conditions, you should consider bypass. If you don't have them, you should avoid it. Countless studies have shown that low-risk patients (i.e., patients without the above conditions) who avoid bypass have as high or higher survival rates than those who undergo bypass under typical hospital conditions. And I believe many low-risk patients could do even better with more aggressive medical therapy.

Significant Blockage of the Left Main Coronary Artery

The left main coronary artery is a short artery, only about an inch long, that divides into the left anterior descending artery coming down the heart wall and the left circumflex branch that goes around to the back of the heart. The left main is rarely affected with plaque buildup, unlike the left anterior descending artery, and the two should not be confused.

If the left main artery is blocked 90 to 95 percent, it cuts off the blood supply to the entire left side of the heart. Although other arteries can sometimes compensate for blockage, a blockage in the left main artery cannot be compensated for by another vessel.

If you have significant blockage (75 percent or more) in the left main artery, you will know you are ill. Exercise will gener-

ANATOMY OF THE HEART

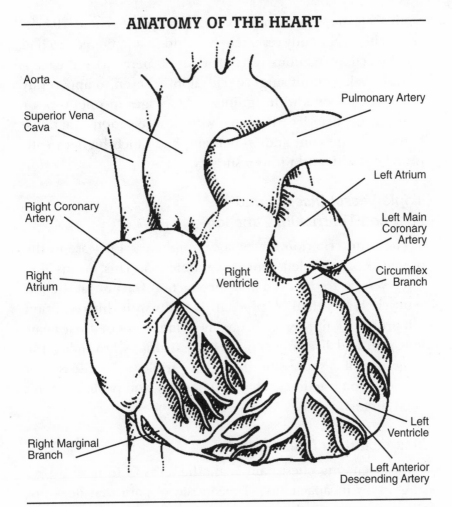

Aorta

Superior Vena Cava

Pulmonary Artery

Left Atrium

Right Coronary Artery

Left Main Coronary Artery

Right Atrium

Right Ventricle

Circumflex Branch

Left Ventricle

Right Marginal Branch

Left Anterior Descending Artery

ally produce angina, noticeable shortness of breath, and changes on the electrocardiogram. Significant blockages of the left main do not occur without signs or symptoms.

Ejection Fraction of Less Than 50 Percent

Your "ejection fraction" is the percentage of blood ejected from your heart with each heartbeat. Healthy hearts have a resting ejection fraction of between 50 percent and 70 percent. The CASS study researchers found that patients who had good ejection fractions (greater than 50 percent) did exceptionally well without surgery. This applied even to apparently quite sick patients with significant blockages in one, two, or even three arteries. Patients with low ejection fractions, between 30 percent and 50 percent, had much higher death rates both with and without surgery.

Triple Vessel Disease and Poor Left Ventricular Function

The third criterion for bypass is triple-vessel disease in the presence of poor left ventricular function. This means that three vessels are blocked and the ejection fraction of the left ventricle is less than 50 percent. Patients with this condition will probably improve their quality of life, increase their heart function, and live longer with bypass surgery, assuming the surgery itself is successful. If you have triple-vessel disease but your ejection fraction is above 50 percent, you probably don't need surgery.

Incapacitating Chest Pain

Incapacitating chest pain is another reason to have bypass surgery. By incapacitating, I mean severe pain that does not respond to medical therapy and limits activity. If you have those symptoms, an angiogram is appropriate to determine where the blockage is located, and bypass surgery may indeed be necessary. If one or more of these problems is present, bypass may improve your quality of life or longevity. But if they are not present, you probably shouldn't have it. Make your decision based on knowledge, not fear.

BAD REASONS FOR BYPASS

Hundreds of thousands of patients submit to bypass even though they don't need it, shouldn't have it, and will be hurt by it. Don't become one of those statistics.

Here are some of the bad reasons for bypass surgery.

Hasty Prognosis

Your doctor says, "Bypass will save your life"—without telling you what kind of heart disease you have.

Bypass surgery is thought to prevent death. But we have seen that it also causes death, and in many patients it does not prevent heart attacks and even promotes heart disease. Bypass can only reduce the risk of death in the extreme cases listed above. Otherwise it is worse than unnecessary—it is dangerous.

But the perception of bypass as an all-around lifesaver persists. Physicians continue to recommend it. Patients continue to submit to it. Insurance companies routinely pay for the operation, whether or not it is actually necessary. Don't be buffaloed. Ask questions. Make them tell you what your real condition is. Find out if you are low or high risk.

Angina—Not a Determinant for Surgery

Angina is a serious condition that requires strict medical supervision. If you have squeezing or pressure-like chest pains you should be under a doctor's supervision. You may even need prescription medication. Angina is created by blockages in or spasms of the coronary arteries that reduce the supply of oxygen to the heart. The pain of angina is your heart's cry for oxygen. Angina is usually symptomatic of heart disease. And it is always painful and scary. Angina, however, is reversible. By following the program I outline later in this book, you can reduce and even eliminate angina.

If you have angina, make sure that your pains are the result of severely blocked arteries before submitting to bypass surgery. Painful arterial spasms can also be caused by stress or nutritional deficiencies. There is also a special type of angina that is not related to plaque buildup. This is called Prinzmetal's variant angina, a disease indicated by coronary artery spasms. It is not brought on by exertion; instead it usually happens when the body is at rest and it can occur at odd times during the day or night. The condition is more common in women under the age of fifty and usually responds to magnesium supplementation.

Stable and Unstable Angina   Perhaps you've heard the terms stable and unstable angina, and do not fully understand what they mean. The difference is basically this: Unstable angina occurs not only with strain, but also at rest, and is generally incapacitating. Stable angina can be very painful and terrifying, but it occurs only when you are exerting yourself.

Hospital admissions for unstable angina have risen from 130,000 in 1983 to 570,000 in 1991. More than 25 percent of these patients end up submitting to invasive heart surgery. This increase in diagnosis of unstable angina, during a period when heart disease is actually decreasing, leads me to suspect that doctors may be expanding their definition of unstable angina in order to operate on more patients.

Many of my patients have been diagnosed by other doctors as having unstable angina when in fact their angina was stable, or it wasn't angina at all. If you are diagnosed as having unstable angina, get a second opinion.

Relief of Nonincapacitating Pain

Many patients who undergo bypass report a reduction in chest pain. Does this mean that their hearts are getting more oxygen?

Not necessarily. Although bypass often does provide more oxygen to the heart, there are other reasons for the relief of angina pains.

In approximately 5 percent of all bypass operations, the surgery itself causes heart attacks. If the heart muscle killed in the attack was the cause of the pain, the pain will go away. This is similar to alleviating the pain of an infected toe by amputation.

Also, the nerves that carry pain messages from the heart are severed during the operation. It would be virtually impossible for anginal pain to be transmitted soon after bypass surgery.

Finally, bypass serves as a placebo. A placebo is a cure that appears to work not because of any genuine healing, but because it persuades patients to believe they are healed. Scientific studies often include placebos like sugar pills to see if the effects of treatment aren't purely psychological. Surgical operations are powerful placebos because of the emotional involvement of the patient, who often feels that something as dramatic and as dangerous as surgery must be a cure.

Whatever does cause the pain relief, it is only temporary. In about 70 percent of all bypass patients, angina returns within five years.

ST-Segment Depression

The medical test that most frequently starts patients on the path to unnecessary heart surgery is the exercise stress test. And ST-segment depression is often the initial indicator for further testing and eventual surgery.

The ST segment is the electrical fingerprint of the heart. If there is damage or lack of oxygen to the heart, the ST segment is flattened or depressed. Prevailing wisdom says that the greater the ST-segment depression, the more evidence there is of heart disease.

A drop in the ST segment is reason for concern, but it's not, by itself, reason to start thinking about surgery. An important study has proven that.

The Lown Group   In 1981, Drs. Bernard Lown, Philip Podrid, and Thomas Graboys from the Harvard School of Public Health conducted a study assessing the results of 212 male patients who showed very significant ST-segment drops on the treadmill.[1]

The participants, thirty-nine to eighty years of age, all had documented coronary artery disease, and bypass surgery had been recommended. All but nine of the patients stayed on a medical treatment regimen. The doctors followed these patients for fifty-nine months. Only 1.4 percent of the patients died (1.3 percent of the patients who submitted to surgery died), leading the researchers to conclude:

"ST-segment depression is not associated with a poor prognosis. There is rarely a need to resort to cardiac surgery: Medical management is highly successful and associated with a low mortality."

"Significant" Heart Disease

What if you're told you have "significant" heart disease?

Dr. Whady Hueb reported in 1989 in the *American Journal of Cardiology* on 150 patients, all of whom had been urged to have bypass surgery and all of whom refused.[2] The group was pretty sick: 58 percent had had a heart attack; 36 percent had unstable angina; 13 percent had had congestive heart failure.

In other words, many of these patients had "significant" heart disease. Yet, without bypass surgery, only six patients died during an eight-year period. These patients were being treated with standard heart drugs—and they improved.

When surgery was recommended, only a total of 11 percent

of the patients were angina-free. By the end of the study, 68.5 percent were angina-free.

In addition, the heart attack rate was surprisingly low in all groups. When bypass was recommended, 60 percent of the patients had suffered a heart attack. After eight years of routine medical heart therapy—and eight years after refusing the bypass—only 10 percent (fifteen patients) had had new heart attacks. Only three were fatal.

The authors concluded:

> The main findings in the present study are the high survival rate, the significant remission of symptoms, and the low incidence of coronary events in medically treated patients with severe CAD (coronary artery disease).

If your doctor tells you that you have "significant" heart disease, ask him to be specific. Have him explain what's really going on instead of hiding behind vague terminology.

Blockage Greater Than 70 Percent In One Vessel

In 1988, Nicholas Danchin and his group at France's University Hospital of Nancy-Braois Department of Cardiology and Cardiovascular Surgery published the results of a study in which they had followed forty-four patients with single-vessel disease for ten years.[3]

The angiograms of ninety-one men showed discrete, well-defined blockages of greater than 70 percent in one coronary artery. Forty-seven of these men, more than half of whom reported significant chest pain, elected to have surgery immediately after their angiogram; forty-four decided to continue with their regular medical treatment. The latter were Danchin's patients.

Those in the group that chose not to have surgery were very

ill. Twenty-one of them had already had heart attacks (compared with nine of the forty-seven who selected surgery). Nine of them had unstable angina; twenty-two had stable angina; fifteen had atypical chest pain and abnormal resting EKG; and eight had ejection fractions of less than 50 percent.

Ten years later forty of the original forty-four men were available for follow-up: Fourteen of them were better, and ten were still at work after ten years.

The researchers concluded that such high survival rates looked like the numbers of a population with normal coronary arteries.

In addition to these favorable survival results, the quality of life for the patients over the ten-year follow-up period was quite satisfactory. Although nearly all the patients were on medical treatment after ten years, the vast majority of them felt well. And they felt that way without undergoing any kind of dangerous, invasive surgery.

These results are not unusual. Dr. Dean Ornish took twenty-four patients with severe cardiovascular disease and isolated them for twenty-four days. He gave them a vegetarian diet with 10 percent of calories from fat and he taught them stress reduction techniques. He compared these with twenty-four control patients who received routine care from their cardiologists.

The results were clear: Simple diet change was a powerful, remarkably beneficial therapy. Dr. Ornish found that his patients increased the amount of time they could sustain exercise by 44 percent; their total work performance increased by 55 percent; ejection fraction from rest to exercise was increased by 6.4 percent; their collective cholesterol count dropped from 229 to 182 in less than a month; and the frequency of angina attacks was reduced by 91 percent.[4]

Second Opinions: Life Savers

Because the need for surgery varies so much from patient to patient, always seek a second opinion. Get the information you need to take control. Information can save your life.

The most important medical article published on second opinions for bypass surgery, "Results of a Second Opinion Program for Coronary Artery Bypass Graft Surgery," *Journal of the American Medical Association,*[5] was written by Dr. Thomas Graboys, a teaching cardiologist at Harvard Medical School.

Thomas Graboys, M.D., of the Lown Cardiovascular Center in Boston, published the center's results on eighty-eight patients, all of whom sought a second opinion from Dr. Graboys and his colleagues when bypass surgery was recommended to them by their local cardiologists.[6] After examining the patients, doctors at the Cardiovascular Center agreed that fourteen should have bypass surgery while seventy-four should not. All told, sixty patients continued on with routine medical heart therapy.

Four years later, all of the sixty patients were alive and well, and only two patients (3.3 percent) had sustained nonfatal heart attacks. Seventy percent of those who refused surgery were actively and fully employed, while only 45 percent of those who had bypass were able to handle their normal work load.

In the same issue of the *Journal of the American Medical Association,* Henry McIntosh, M.D., past president of the American College of Cardiology, wrote an editorial supporting this systematic approach to getting second opinions when bypass surgery is recommended.[7]

Graboys and his colleagues (known as the Lown group) have devised a five-step checklist to help heart patients determine the degree of cardiac risk they might be facing:

—————————— **CHECKLIST FOR SURGERY** ——————————

If you "check out" on each of the following five points you should be able to avoid heart surgery:

_____ Your left ventricle isn't impaired or damaged, and your ejection fraction is more than 50 percent.

_____ There are other causes for your angina that could be remedied without surgery.

_____ An extensive treadmill exercise stress test does not show exercise-induced arrhythmias.

_____ It is possible to institute a nonsurgical therapy program.

_____ You do not have a greater than 70 percent blockage in the left main coronary artery.

Get a copy of the article from your local library and take it to your doctor's office. Together you can determine whether you meet the Lown group criteria.

Finding a Doctor for a Second Opinion

Don't ask your doctor to recommend a physician for your second opinion. Contact an entirely new physician, one who doesn't know your regular doctor. Or ask for referrals from the American College of Advancement in Medicine (the address is ACAM P.O. Box 3427, Laguna Hills, CA 92653), or a local referral service. Ask for a doctor who deals in preventive medicine, with a specialty in cardiovascular diseases. Call the doctor and talk to him about his methods for coming up with a second opinion. Compare them with the Lown group guidelines. If his are similar, make an appointment.

Facts Not Fear

Giving second opinions to patients who have had heart surgery recommended to them has been a major part of my medical practice for over fifteen years. I see patients all the time who are scared, confused, and ill-informed. And I try to empower them by telling them the truth about their condition and helping them make their own decision. Usually they choose not to have surgery—almost always the right decision.

I steer most people away from heart surgery, not because I am against all surgery, but because the nonsurgical approach is usually the safest and most effective course to take. Remember, patients who are true candidates for bypass surgery are those who have a severe blockage in the left main artery, severe incapacitating chest pain not controllable by medicines, an ejection fraction of less than 50 percent, or three vessels blocked with decreased left venticular function.

I then encourage the patient to return to the original physician and discuss the second opinion and the scientific studies that support it. Then I ask that he or she consider the options once again. A decision to have surgery should be made by a well-informed patient, not someone terrified beyond all reason.

CHAPTER FOUR

Angiograms: Slippery Slope To Surgery

Neither safe nor effective.
Better, safer tests you should have first.
The right time to have an angiogram.

The angiogram is called a diagnostic test. But as currently used by heart doctors, it is an invasive and potentially dangerous procedure that is used as a prelude to even more invasive and even more dangerous surgery.

WHAT IS AN ANGIOGRAM?

To perform an angiogram, a doctor inserts a catheter into the artery of the leg, usually in the groin, then threads the catheter back up toward the heart. When it reaches the small openings that lead off to the two main arteries of the heart, the doctor injects a contrast dye and takes a series of X-ray pictures. The pictures reveal kinks, constrictions, and irregularities in the arterial system, usually identified as cholesterol blockages. It is a long, uncomfortable procedure that costs more than $1,000 and requires at least a day's hospitalization.

The angiogram has become the gold standard for testing heart patients. It is done more than a million times a year, and many cardiologists say it is the only truly definitive test that assesses heart function. This belief lends itself to two inappropriate uses of the angiogram.

The first inappropriate use is when physicians use angiograms as an initial test, ignoring the less expensive and far less dangerous noninvasive procedures. The second inappropriate use is when patients are subjected to an angiogram even when all of the noninvasive tests reveal that heart disease is not present. Angiograms should be conducted only when other methods have indicated that severe blockages exist.

The very creation of the angiogram was a fluke. In the mid-1960s, a doctor accidentally squirted dye into one of his patient's small heart arteries. He expected his mistake would kill the patient, but instead it revealed cholesterol obstruction of the artery.

The angiogram business was off and running. And the concept of actually treating heart disease was left behind.

ARE ANGIOGRAMS SAFE?

There are two ways in which angiograms can harm you. First, the procedure itself can cause damage. Second, the test can push you toward unnecessary and dangerous surgery.

Your doctor may never tell you this, but an angiogram can trigger a heart attack or stroke that could kill you. The death rate is low, usually less than 1 percent. But is a diagnostic test worth that kind of risk?

Angiograms can also cause nonfatal heart attacks and

strokes. And the catheter can damage the walls of the arteries it travels through, causing hardening of the arteries.

But the greater risk is that the angiogram will be successful—that is, the test will show coronary disease and your cardiologist will start pushing surgery on you. An angiogram is often the first step on the road toward unnecessary surgery.

ARE ANGIOGRAMS ACCURATE?

The National Heart, Lung, and Blood Institute conducted a study[1] in which three arteriographers, specialists in interpreting the procedure, read angiograms taken from twenty-eight deceased patients before they died. When their readings were compared with autopsy findings, 82 percent of the angiograms were found to be inaccurate.

In the second part of the study, thirty of the angiogram films were given to radiologists at three separate medical centers. Thirty-eight percent of the time the radiologists came up with different interpretations of the angiograms.

In the third and last leg of the study, the same thirty films were recirculated to the first group of arteriographers who were unaware they were viewing films they had seen before. This time they not only disagreed with each other, they disagreed with their own initial readings. In 32 percent of the cases, their second evaluations differed from their first.

Interobserver Variability

What would happen if you built a home in which the architect had his opinion of what an inch meant, and the contractor and carpenter each had his own differing opinion?

It happens in medicine all the time, and no one seems to be bothered by it. "Interobserver variability," as they call it when two experts get different readings from the same test, is a concept so twisted that only doctors could have come up with it. And it has plagued angiograms from the beginning.

Dr. Leonard M. Zir of Massachusetts General Hospital compared the readings of four experienced angiographers reading twenty consecutive angiograms. These angiographers had been working together as a group for years and had led many patients toward heart surgery. But when Dr. Zir had them read angiograms on their own, he found that their interpretations varied widely.

His study, published in 1976 in *Circulation*,[2] concluded that there was a substantial degree of interobserver variability among even very experienced angiographers. He wrote, "Interobserver variability in the interpretation of lesions in the coronary vessels might be similarly translated into different decisions about the necessity for coronary artery bypass surgery or, if coronary artery bypass surgery is to be performed, which vessels are bypassable. Interobserver variability is a significant limitation of coronary angiography. . . ."

Many of my patients have gotten several different readings on their angiograms. What is interesting is that most patients will give more credibility to the latest reading and never question the accuracy of the test itself.

Angiograms Don't Read Blood Flow Properly

Even an accurate reading of an angiogram may not tell you what you really need to know.

Angiograms show blockages as lumps or bumps in the arteries. But most plaque accumulation is diffuse, with smooth layers of cholesterol buildup lining the artery walls. The angiogram cannot point out this gradual blockage, only abrupt obstructions.

In an angiogram, we see the artery, and the dye inside it represents how much blood is passing through the artery. But we're looking at the length of the artery, not inside. To see how much of the interior of the artery is actually obstructed we would need a cross-sectional view.

Moreover the percentage of an artery that is blocked does not necessarily correlate to the percentage of blood flow through that artery, especially when the blockage is nonsevere. A 50 percent blockage does not produce a 50 percent reduction in blood flow. How much blood is flowing over a 50 percent blockage? One hundred percent! Try putting your thumb over the opening of a running garden hose. Although you cover the hole by 50 percent or more, the same amount of water squirts out, just a little more forcefully.

You have to block the hole off by about 75 percent before there is any reduction in the actual volume of flow. It's a law of fluid dynamics. In the same way, nonsevere blockage does not interfere with blood flow.

In an article in the *New England Journal of Medicine*, researchers Carl W. White, M.D., et al. reported that they had measured blood flow over blockages in thirty-nine patients in an attempt to get a reliable estimate of blood flow from point A to point B.[3] Their results proved that angiograms, while showing arterial blockage, do not reveal how much is flowing. The researchers concluded: "The physiologic effects of the majority of coronary obstructions cannot be determined accurately by conventional angiographic approaches."

The article was accompanied by an editorial which concluded that the results of the White study and others like it "should be profoundly disturbing to all physicians" who have relied on the coronary angiogram to give accurate information about the physiological consequences of individual blockages.

What has been the effect of this study? In 1980 there were 380,000 angiograms performed. In 1994, there were more than a million. Each angiogram performed can be the first step on a slippery slope to unnecessary heart surgery. An angiogram is not a good test for determining if heart surgery is necessary because although it can locate blockages it often cannot show how severe or significant they are.

ALTERNATIVES TO ANGIOGRAPHY

As many as half of all angiograms are unnecessary.

In a study published in the *Journal of the American Medical Association* in 1992, researchers concluded, "In a large fraction of medically stable patients with coronary disease who are urged to undergo coronary angiography, the procedure can be safely deferred. While there may be a limitation in terms of generalizing this experience to all patients with coronary disease, we reasonably conclude that an estimated 50 percent of coronary angiography currently being undertaken in the United States is unnecessary, or at least could be postponed."[4]

Why are angiograms unnecessary? Simple. There are safer, better diagnostic tests that you can take to determine the extent of your heart disease. Don't let yourself be pushed into getting an angiogram if you have not first learned as much as you can from noninvasive tests. Here is a quick introduction to cardiac diagnostic tests currently being used:

Electrocardiogram (EKG)

The EKG is a simple and routine test that is used millions of times every year. It is noninvasive and entails no direct risk to the patient.

Electrodes are attached to the patient's arms, legs, and chest. While the patient lies still, they measure and record the electrical activity of the heart, which is printed out in the form of a series of waves representing each heartbeat.

These waves are broken into segments designated by the letters P, Q, R, S, and T. Each segment represents a different stage of the contraction and relaxation of the heart. P stands for right atrium contraction, QRS represent the contraction of the ventricles, and the T wave shows the relaxation phase of the heartbeat.

While some doctors believe that a flattening or depression of the ST segment indicates damage to the heart muscle, we have already seen how this criterion is being used to push comparatively healthy patients into surgery.

Stress Test

The stress test is basically an EKG that is taken while the patient walks on a treadmill or rides a stationary bicycle. It is used to determine your heart's fitness.

The patient exercises to create a greater level of stress on the heart. Sometimes exercise can induce symptoms like angina. The risk of a fatal heart attack is extremely low, but it has been known to happen. Many patients with severe heart disease are unable to finish the test because of the accompanying pain.

The stress test is easy and relatively safe. Unfortunately, it is sometimes inaccurate, with a high rate of false positives (indicating that heart disease is present when in fact it is not), especially among young women. And there are high false negatives (where heart disease is present but undetected), especially in young men.

Holter Monitoring

A Holter monitor is basically a portable EKG that a patient wears under his clothing for a twenty-four hour period to record the heart's rhythms throughout the day. Holter monitors are safe, but they don't tell you much about blockages in the coronary arteries.

Echocardiography

Echocardiograms are obtained by reflecting high-frequency sounds off various structures in the heart and then translating those sound waves into images. They measure heart size, function, and thickness of the heart muscle and can be used to measure blood flow through the heart chambers. Echocardiograms are noninvasive and very reliable. There is no pain and no risk.

PET Scan

Positron emission tomography (PET), a form of nuclear imaging similar to the CAT scan, measures the heart's metabolism as well as blood flow. A PET scan costs about $1,500, which may sound expensive, but isn't much more than an angiogram, and it's much more accurate, not to mention safer. Despite its proven record, the PET scan has yet to be accepted by the medical establishment.

Thallium Stress Test

In the thallium stress test a small amount of thallium is administered intravenously while you are exercising. Then you stop exercising and are put beneath a scanning camera. By this time the thallium is concentrated in your heart, where it is picked up by the camera. Unfortunately, the test is notoriously inaccurate, incorrectly identifying nearly half the regions with decreased blood supply as irreversibly damaged. That's all some doctors need to scare you into surgery.

Ejection Fraction

The ejection fraction is a simple measure of heart health. It has nothing to do with blockages, pain, or other aspects of heart disease. It is always included as part of the angiogram test, but it can also be determined by the echocardiogram or simply by a conversation between doctor and patient.

The normal heart pumps out 50 to 75 percent of the blood contained in the chambers with each stroke. For instance, if the heart at rest fills with blood to a capacity of 100 cc and the next stroke pumps out 70 cc, then the ejection fraction is 70 percent. If it fills with 100 cc and pumps out 35 cc, the ejection fraction is 35 percent. Healthy hearts will have a higher ejection fraction than unhealthy hearts because they are stronger, less dilated, and more efficient.

The five-year CASS study demonstrated that patients with ejection fractions of 50 percent or greater, whether they had a one-, two-, or three-vessel disease, had exactly the same death rate as those in the medical group who did not have surgery— about 1 percent a year.

At the ten-year CASS follow-up of the patients with an ejection fraction of 50 percent, those patients who did not have surgery actually had fewer heart attacks than those who had surgery.

Using the ejection fraction a responsible physician can identify patients who, even though they appear sick, are better off avoiding surgery. There is no excuse not to use this test. A physician can usually estimate the ejection fraction simply by talking to the patient—most patients with normal ejection fractions have no history of heart attacks, swelling, or frequent shortness of breath. Most patients with poor ejection fractions have had heart attacks in the past that have weakened the heart or eliminated sections of the heart muscle.

WHAT ARE ANGIOGRAMS GOOD FOR?

Basically angiograms are useful when you have already decided to have surgery or other invasive procedures.

Angiogram readings are good road maps for such procedures. If surgery is necessary, then the diseased areas of the arteries have to be pinpointed. Angiograms can help do that. But they shouldn't be used as an initial diagnostic tool. Use safer and more accurate methods first.

If, after you've undergone the noninvasive tests like the stress test and echocardiogram, you still need to know more about your arterial blockages, then you might want to consider an angiogram. But be careful, and don't let the doctors use it as a scare tactic to get you under the knife. Remember my criteria for bypass surgery and use the angiogram to help determine if your case is that extreme.

CHAPTER FIVE

Angioplasty: Two Steps Backward

Why cardiologists love this dangerous procedure, how it causes heart disease, and why you should just say no.

Kailash Mehta had no symptoms of heart disease. She seemed fine until a routine test revealed a blockage in one of her coronary arteries. Her doctors recommended that she undergo angioplasty, a procedure in which a balloon is expanded inside a coronary artery in order to push plaque aside and reopen clogged arteries (more about this later). She agreed and signed a consent form. The doctors assured her that the procedure was safe.

She went into the angioplasty lab and lay down on the table. The cardiologist tried three times to clear the blockage. On the third try, the artery burst. Kailash was rushed into surgery for an emergency bypass. But it was already too late. Heart failure had caused brain damage. She went into a coma. After nine weeks she died.[1]

This story is tragic, but not uncommon.

Kailash was a victim of something called *iatrogenesis,* a fancy word for saying that her illness, and eventual death, was caused by her doctor. It's something like a war injury from the "friendly fire" of your own troops.

NEITHER SAFE NOR SIMPLE

Angioplasty, also called balloon angioplasty (the technical term is percutaneous transluminal coronary angioplasty or PTCA), is a procedure in which a catheter is inserted into an artery in the groin, as is done in an angiogram. But unlike the angiogram, this catheter snakes all the way into the coronary arteries themselves. When it reaches a blockage, a balloon is inflated to crush the surrounding plaque and expand the artery to increase blood flow to the heart. This is done under local anesthesia and the patient usually spends one night in the hospital.

But angioplasty is not as simple as it's made to sound, and it certainly isn't safe. As we have seen in the case of Kailash Mehta, angioplasty can kill you. The catheter can rupture the artery, resulting in hemorrhage and heart failure. It can also cause a fatal heart attack or stroke. The death rate for angioplasty ranges from 2 to 4 percent, depending on which hospital you go to. And there's another 5 percent chance that you will need emergency bypass surgery as the result of an angioplasty.

There are numerous other possible—or probable—side effects from angioplasty, including damage to the arteries, blood clots, increased plaque deposits, and reclosure of the clogged artery. Angioplasty damages arterial walls, which sets the stage for reclosure that is often more rapid and severe than would be expected from normal plaque buildup. Arteries that have been treated with angioplasty reclose at a rate of 35 percent within six months. And patients who undergo angioplasty have a greater likelihood of future surgery than those who avoid it.

Angioplasty is a dangerous procedure with a high risk of side effects. What benefits angioplasty does provide are often short lived. And because of the damage to the arteries that occurs even in "successful" procedures, angioplasty creates more heart disease.

THE ANGIOPLASTY INDUSTRY

Angioplasty got its start when the *New England Journal of Medicine* showcased the procedure in an article by Andreas R. Greuntzig, the inventor of angioplasty.[2]

The article related Dr. Greuntzig's experience of inflating a balloon inside the coronary arteries of fifty patients over an eighteen-month period. It stated that "this technique was used in human beings after preliminary trials in dogs and cadavers," as if such information would assure us of the procedure's safety. Though Dr. Greuntzig was excited by the results, dangers were there from the beginning:

> ➤ The treatment group had a 4 percent annual mortality rate.

> ➤ Fourteen percent of the patients had to undergo emergency bypass surgery.

> ➤ Six percent underwent repeat angioplasties because the first procedure was not successful.

It is not uncommon for new procedures to have initial difficulties. That's why we have studies and tests, and usually the results improve, or the procedure is modified or discontinued. But in the case of angioplasty, although the results didn't improve, the procedure became immensely popular. Angioplasty was unknown before 1979. In 1983 there were 30,000 angioplasties. In 1993 there were 400,000. As in the case of bypass, this phenomenal growth occurred at a time when the rate of heart disease was actually declining.

CARDIOLOGISTS ARE NOW SURGEONS TOO

One of the reasons angioplasty enjoys such popularity is that it is enormously profitable. And since you don't have to be a surgeon to perform angioplasty, cardiologists have become its greatest proponents. As a result, angioplasty has changed the very structure of the cardiac profession.

Prior to angioplasty, the cardiologist—who is a medical heart specialist, not a surgeon—was in the patient's corner as an advocate and adviser. The cardiologist had no financial incentive to recommend surgery; his advice to patients was expert and disinterested.

Thanks to angioplasty, however, cardiologists have become "surgeons." They now evaluate the patient, recommend treatment, and then perform the angioplasty themselves.

For cardiologists, angioplasty is a gold mine. At an average cost of $15,000, angioplasty is cheaper than bypass, but it still makes a great profit for both doctor and hospital. Right now it's a $6 billion industry. And the average cardiologist makes almost $200,000 a year.

That's the financial cost of angioplasty. But what's the human cost? A conservative estimate of angioplasty's mortality rate is 2 percent, which means thousands of deaths per year. The pain and suffering, emergency and repeat operations, and deaths due to accelerated heart disease that angioplasty directly causes are inestimable.

COMPLICATIONS OF ANGIOPLASTY

The major coronary arteries are no larger than a pencil. When artery walls are injured, fatty deposits form and are soon joined by other substances, including calcium, which makes the arteries sclerotic—that is, hard and rigid. Angioplasty is an attempt to push the plaque aside, allowing freer blood flow. But for many angioplasty patients, the procedure is more dangerous than their relatively low-risk heart disease.

The risk of death increases with age. One study found the death rate from angioplasty in Medicare patients was 3.9 percent, roughly one in twenty-five patients. The complication rate was 13.5 percent.

These complications are often associated with the damage done by the procedure to the coronary arteries. Since heart disease starts when the arterial walls are damaged (this will be discussed in depth in a later chapter), angioplasty causes further plaque formation. When the catheter is inserted and the balloon is expanded, it nicks and stretches the once smooth artery walls, separating the endothelial cells and letting plaque formations fill in and build, or grow bigger if they already exist.

Dr. Edward Diethrich, M.D., director of the Arizona Heart Institute, used the angioscope, which functions like a miniature periscope, to look at the results of angioplasty. He said that if you look down the artery with an angioscope you will see the real results of an angioplasty and it can look like a war zone.[3]

Numerous other studies have proven that significant arterial damage is caused by angioplasty, including a recent study published in the *Journal of the American College of Cardiology*.[4]

Restenosis

Restenosis is the clinical term for reclosure of an artery. The rate of reclosure in angioplasty is scandalous. More than a third of treated arteries close up within six months. That's a 33 percent failure rate. And despite desperate efforts, angioplasty proponents have failed miserably to bring down the reclosure rates.

In the cover story of *Medical World News* in February 1991, Charles D. Bankhead wrote, "Angioplasters have yet to slay their major nemesis: restenosis. That dragon continues to rear its head as vengefully as it did when Swiss cardiologist Andreas Greuntzig first dilated a coronary vessel. Restenosis has defied every mechanical and pharmacological assault cardiologists have mounted against the vessel reclosure that occurs in about 40 percent of patients."

In the same story, Spencer King, director of the Greuntzig Cardiovascular Center at Emory University in Atlanta, said, "There is very little the clinician can do right now to prevent restenosis. Prevention efforts are totally 'seat of the pants.'" He continued, "There is no guidance. Everybody is sort of floundering around."[5]

This floundering around has produced an alarming array of devices and techniques that only make the situation more dangerous for the angioplasty patient.

The Stent

What happens when a procedure becomes popular and profitable, even though it doesn't work? The medical establishment will go to great lengths trying to fix it.

When it became apparent that between 20 percent and 40 percent of arteries opened by balloon angioplasty were closing during the first year, there was a technological rush to solve the problem.

One attempt was something called a "stent," a small piece of coiled wire that resembles the spring inside a ballpoint pen. The stent is inserted inside the artery just after the angioplasty balloon has expanded and the artery is open. It is supposed to keep the artery from closing back up.

You might think that putting a small metal spring inside one of your coronary arteries is not a very good idea. Well, you'd be right. The first problem that emerged was that stents were found to attract blood clots and form blockages inside the artery. In initial studies, reclosure was found in 20 percent of patients. To remedy that, doctors started prescribing anticlotting drugs to their patients with stents. The result was bleeding complications in about 10 percent of all patients.

A study published in the *American Journal of Cardiology* found significant bleeding and damage in 16.8 percent of stenting procedures.[6] The researchers concluded: "The overall risk of vascular complications with new device procedures (stenting, directional atherectomy) is greater than that traditionally seen with balloon angioplasty alone...."

As if the risks of angioplasty weren't bad enough, now we have stents to worry about. But that's not all, scientists have now come up with a rotorooter for the heart called atherectomy.

A ROTOROOTER FOR THE HEART

In 1987 the first coronary atherectomy was performed. The atherectomy is similar to angioplasty, except that plaque is drilled away.

There are two different kinds of atherectomy. Directional atherectomy is the most widely used procedure. It uses a catheter with a rotating blade at its end. The blade shaves the plaque blocking the coronary artery. Of course, the blade shaves the artery as well, creating nicks and cuts throughout the artery and seriously damaging the artery walls.

The other is called rotational atherectomy, which uses a high-speed, rotating, diamond-chip burr tip to pulverize obstructions. These particles then pass through the blood-stream, possibly causing clots.

Given the track record of angioplasty, it's not surprising that atherectomy is dangerous, ineffective, and promotes heart disease. The whirling blades of the atherectomy device cut away at the artery walls, creating the damage that makes heart disease possible in the first place.

A study published in the *New England Journal of Medicine* examined atherectomy patients and found that six months later the atherectomy reclosure rate was 50 percent. However, the truly astounding statistic was the six-month death rate: 8.6 percent (one out of twelve).[7]

BYPASS VS. ANGIOPLASTY, THE SHOWDOWN

From its inception, angioplasty has been touted as a low-cost, low-risk alternative to bypass. Though it may cost about half as much as bypass, it certainly cannot be considered low risk. But has it supplanted bypass?

Not at all. In 1983, when angioplasty was in its infancy, there were 180,000 bypass operations. Ten years later, angioplasty had increased to 400,000 operations, about the same number as bypass operations.

In fact, angioplasty and bypass are being performed repeatedly on the same patients. Sometimes an angioplasty goes wrong and the patient must have a bypass. More often though, angioplasty must be repeated because the blockages come back. As Dr. William Castelli, head of the prestigious Framingham Heart Study, says, "Angioplasty is like a potato chip. You can't have just one."[8]

In October 1994, two major studies involving more than 750 patients and comparing bypass surgery and angioplasty were published in the *New England Journal of Medicine*.[9] One was done at my alma mater, Emory University, the other in Germany.

In both studies bypass patients were more likely to have heart attacks than angioplasty patients. In the angioplasty group, the most frequent complication was emergency bypass surgery. In the Emory study 10 percent of the angioplasty patients required emergency bypass surgery!

The German study lasted one year, after which the combined death and heart attack rate was 13.6 percent in the bypass group and 6 percent in the angioplasty group. Almost half of the angioplasty patients had to be worked on again within one year!

In the Emory study 14 percent of the bypass patients and 63 percent of the angioplasty patients required a repeat procedure within three years.

These studies received wide play in the press, with the general conclusion that angioplasty was a safer, cheaper alternative to bypass surgery. Conspicuously lacking from these studies, however, was a control group of patients who received neither bypass surgery nor angioplasty, but pursued a course of conservative, noninvasive treatment. They would have been hands-down winners in safety, mortality, cost, and improved health.

DON'T LET IT HAPPEN TO YOU

In the past few years, cardiovascular residents have been taking a third year of training to gain experience in catheterization or angioplasty, which increases their marketability. The resulting abundance of practitioners means that many will perform the procedure on patients who don't need it. To a man with a hammer, everything looks like a nail. And to some cardiologists with catheters, every patient needs an angioplasty.

Since heart disease is declining, thanks in part to the growing popularity of noninvasive therapies like The Whitaker Wellness Program, the number of patients who could truly benefit from aggressive intervention is also declining. Medical practitioners are therefore behaving like entrepreneurs, seeking out and acquiring new patients.

As part of this new "marketing strategy," EKGs and stress tests are often offered at a very low cost by hospitals. They may seem like a good deal. But those screening devices are often used to find potential patients and funnel them into bypass or angioplasty.

As a result even patients who are not sick can find themselves being wheeled into the operating room.

An angioplasty is an operation. If your doctor says you need one, get a second opinion.

CHAPTER SIX

Women and Heart Surgery

The special dangers of bypass and angioplasty for women and what they can do to protect themselves.

Three-quarters of all bypass operations are performed on men. That's actually good news, since women run a much greater risk from the surgery than men. They are twice as likely to die during bypass and face far greater complications. Researchers have known for years about this higher risk and for a long time thought it was because the women who underwent bypass were more sick than men, which is often the case. But a new study has shown that women are at greater risk because their bodies, and therefore their arteries, are on average smaller than men's. And it's much more dangerous to operate on smaller arteries.

The study, conducted by the Northern New England Cardiovascular Study Group, looked at patients who had bypass surgery in five different hospitals in northern New England.[1]

They reported that of the 132 patients who died, 3.2 percent of them were men and 7.3 percent were women. They also found that smaller men had a higher risk of perioperative death (death during or soon after surgery), again due to the size of their arteries.

This doubling of the death risk in women was mirrored in another study. Cedars-Sinai Medical Center in Los Angeles found that the death rate for women who had bypass was 4.6 percent, while only 2.8 percent of men died from the surgery.[2]

Other studies have shown a higher failure rate of bypass in women, and a greater risk of reoperation. Since a second or third operation requires longer operating time because the intial grafts have to be removed first, bleeding may be more profuse.

Women should be extremely careful in deciding whether to undergo bypass. The risks are much greater and the potential benefits far less.

WOMEN AND ANGIOGRAMS

Women do not get angiograms as frequently as men. The Cedars-Sinai study referred to above showed that while 40 percent of men get angiograms after indication of an abnormal heartbeat during a stress test, only 4 percent of women get catheterized.

While the angiogram is overused and is often the first step to unnecessary heart disease, this study is troubling because it is yet another indication that cardiologists don't seem to be paying the same attention to equal symptoms among men and women. They still think of heart disease as a predominantly male disease.

Moreover, men have angiograms at a rate ten times higher than women but have bypass at a rate only three times higher, which indicates that once women do get catheterized, they are more likely to go into surgery. Women are not diagnosed as aggressively as men, so only the sickest women actually get tested. Then they are pushed into surgery.

If you are a woman about to undergo diagnostic tests for heart disease, don't insist on an angiogram just to be one of the boys. But do go into the tests knowing what symptoms to look for and what questions to ask your doctor. Insist on exhaustive noninvasive tests, especially an echocardiogram. Have the doctor discuss the results with you in detail. In short: Don't let yourself be steered into unnecessary surgery, but don't let your doctor disregard your symptoms either.

WOMEN AND ANGIOPLASTY

Women also run a significantly higher risk from angioplasty. According to a study by the National Heart, Lung, and Blood Institute, women who have angioplasty are ten times more likely to die from it than men.[3] The institute studied sixteen medical centers across the country, and although only one-quarter of the patients were women, fourteen of the eighteen patients who died were women, and twelve of those fourteen were over the age of sixty-five.

Age may explain about half of these deaths, according to the study. But the higher risk of both death and complications probably also has to do with women's smaller arteries. This is because the catheter can rupture an artery, causing fatal hemorrhage or heart attack. Thus angioplasty is far riskier for women than for men.

In light of the report, the American Heart Association said, "Women may want to think twice before asking for 'equal treatment' from their heart doctors."[4]

THE YENTL SYNDROME

Nearly half of all who die from heart disease are women. True, men run a slightly greater risk of developing heart disease. But heart disease is much more dangerous for women, because women who have a heart attack are more likely to die from it than men.

Women are increasingly prone to heart disease after menopause. The older they get, the greater the risk. By age forty-five, heart disease affects one out of nine women. By age sixty-four that ratio has increased to one out of three. Since symptoms of heart disease in women tend to be less dramatic than in men, the disease often goes unnoticed until it has done significant damage. Doctors haven't helped any by ignoring their female patients until they become very sick, and then overtreating them.

Two major studies in the *New England Journal of Medicine* provoked a huge debate on the role of bias in diagnosing and treating women with heart disease.[5] The studies looked at more than 85,000 heart patients and found that women were not being treated as aggressively as men. That is, although they showed similar symptoms of angina, they did not get tested as frequently as men.

Dr. Bernadine Healy, director of the National Institutes of Health, who wrote the accompanying editorial, called the less attentive care for women "the Yentl syndrome" after the movie in which the heroine had to disguise herself as a man in order to attend school to study the Talmud.

But another study by Dr. Thomas Graboys showed that while men were twice as likely to undergo one of the invasive cardiac procedures as women, bypass was performed with equal frequency among both men and women who had a angiogram.[6] So while women are not treated as aggressively in the initial diagnostic phase, once it is established that they have heart disease, they are treated much more aggressively than men.

If women are not tested as aggressively as men—which the previously mentioned studies and my own anecdotal evidence seem to support—then they are lucky.

But once women are diagnosed as having heart disease, their doctors pursue more aggressive treatment than they do with their male patients. Male doctors must still think that women are the weaker vessel and unable to make decisions about their own bodies. Prove the doctors wrong. Don't give in to the heart surgery trap.

CHAPTER SEVEN

Money And Medicine

Why a country with less and less heart disease has more and more heart surgery.

Heart surgery rarely works. Yet it's more popular than ever. Why is the heart surgery industry booming? Because it means big bucks for doctors, hospitals, and surgical supply companies. Approximately $25 billion a year is spent on the three major operations (bypass, angioplasty, and atherectomy) alone. Before the surgery boom, doctors couldn't do much about heart disease, except give their patients nitroglycerin and hope they would stick to their new diets. Then bypass came along and all of a sudden heart surgery became big business.

THE BYPASS BOOM

When first introduced, bypass was successful with patients who had extreme symptoms. Soon, doctors began to ask whether the surgery could be used for patients with less severe conditions. When the medical evidence came in, the three major studies—VACS (Veterans Administration Cooperative Study), CASS (Coronary Artery Surgery Study), and Euro-CASS (the European Coronary Artery Surgery Study)—all proved that only very sick patients, patients with left main blockage, or three-vessel disease with impaired ventricular function, benefited from bypass (see chapter 2).

Even the seriously ill patients who did get some good from bypass still suffered the same rate of nonfatal heart attacks. Their angina not only returned as the grafted arteries began to close, but they were hospitalized more often than those who did not undergo surgery. Even "successful" grafts closed after five to seven years.

Despite the scientific evidence that bypass surgery helped, to a limited extent, only high-risk patients, the procedure began to be used on low-risk patients as well.

At the Crossroads

In the same issue of the *New England Journal of Medicine* in which the VACS study appeared, Dr. Eugene Braunwald of Harvard wrote an editorial titled "Coronary-Artery Surgery at the Crossroads." Dr. Braunwald observed with alarm that "what might be considered an 'industry' is being built around this operation.... This rapidly growing enterprise is developing a momentum and constituency of its own, and as time passes, it will be progressively more difficult and costly to curtail it materially."[1]

That's exactly what has happened. The growth of bypass surgery has been phenomenal. In 1971, 21,000 bypass operations were performed. By 1979 that number had increased fivefold, to approximately 100,000. Since then, the operation has increased by almost 400 percent. In 1991, 407,000 bypass operations were performed.[2]

More Doctors, More Surgery

The growth of bypass surgery reflects not an increase in heart disease, but an increase in doctors.

Before bypass surgery was developed, many heart surgeons were underemployed. Then bypass came along and quickly provided a virtually unlimited source of clients.

Over the past forty years Americans have grown appreciably healthier in many ways. Predictably these decades have seen a measurable drop in the death rate from cardiovascular disease, a lessening of the severity of symptoms, and an improvement in the cardiovascular health of the nation at large. The death rate from heart disease in 1950 was 355 per 100,000. By 1990 it had dropped to 289 per 100,000.[3] (Lest you think that this decline is due to surgical pratices, remember what the three major studies showed: that surgery only extends longevity in a few, high-risk patients. And it never cures heart disease.)

Yet as heart disease decreased, surgery increased. This increase in surgeries has nothing to do with the health of the hearts of Americans and has a lot to do with the wealth of doctors and hospitals. There are now more than 16,000 cardiologists making an average of almost $200,000 a year. (Compare that to the average family practitioner who makes $102,660.) The average bypass surgery costs $40,000. Multiply that times 400,000 procedures and you've got a $16 billion industry. All told, invasive heart surgery is worth some $25 billion a year.

Despite the obvious and well-documented risks of reoperation (discussed in a previous chapter), the rate of reoperation continues to grow. More and more patients are going in for second operations, up from 2.5 percent a year in 1981 to 7.7 percent per year in 1991.[4] What do you do when you try something and it doesn't work? If you're a heart surgeon, you try it again.

Easy Money

Operating a cardiac care unit is like having a license to print money. Given the third-party payer system that prevails in health care today, the hospital is generously reimbursed no matter how dubious the benefits of bypass surgery.

Just how important is money in determining what kind of coronary care you will get? If you're uninsured, you're 39 percent less likely to get an angiogram than an insured patient and 29 percent less likely to undergo bypass—Medicaid sometimes picks up the check for that.[5]

The heart surgeon is seen as the star of the hospital, performing risky operations at high visibility. And heart surgery is extremely profitable, especially compared with other procedures. According to the Advisory Board Company, a consulting firm based in Washington, D.C., nearly 25 percent of all hospital revenues come from cardiology-related business.[6] The big four procedures—angiograms, angioplasty, bypass surgery, and heart-valve surgery—make up 80 percent of that business. The profit margins on heart surgery are substantial. Angiograms make a 70 percent profit, bypass makes 40 percent, and angioplasty about 37 percent. And heart surgeons bring in $11,000 per patient, the highest rate of any specialty and more than twice as much as the average doctor.[7]

What is behind these extraordinary profits? For one thing, some very questionable conflicts of interest. As the *Journal of the American Medical Association* put it, all too often "the same physician who decides whether a diagnostic or therapeutic procedure is to be done is... also the one who does the procedure, interprets the findings," decides on additional procedures, "and is paid for each step of the way."[8]

Consumer Reports pointed out the following examples of the troubling relationship between cardiac care and profits:

"A study of pacemaker implantations in Philadelphia found that 20 percent were unnecessary and 36 percent were problematic.

"A San Diego team found that, among patients who had been hospitalized with mild heart attacks, 40 percent of those who got angiograms didn't need them."[9]

The magazine told the story of how the rate of heart surgery doubled in Manchester, New Hampshire, once the city got its own cardiac center. More than half of the bypasses performed at the new center, moreover, were on very low risk patients.

Once the technology is in place, it is going to be used, whether it is needed or not.

Approximately one million Americans are stricken with angina each year. More than 550,000 patients are treated with either bypass or angioplasty or both. That means that more than half of those diagnosed with angina submit to some form of invasive surgery.

That's too many victims.

The Real Causes of Heart Disease

PART TWO

The Real Cause
of Heart Disease

CHAPTER EIGHT

What Is Heart Disease?

Understand the two-step process of heart disease and you will be on the way toward healing yourself.

O ne million Americans will die this year, victims of the Great American Lifestyle. We don't exercise enough. We don't get proper nutrition. We eat too many animal fats. And we believe the medical establishment when it tells us that little can be done about heart disease except surgery.

Heart disease is seen as a natural cause of death. It is not. It is an illness that in most cases could have been prevented. If you don't want heart disease, you can avoid it. If you have heart disease, you can reverse it. But the first step is to understand what heart disease is and how it gets started.

WHAT IS HEART DISEASE?

Heart disease is something of a misnomer. In most cases,

there's nothing really wrong with your heart. It's your arteries that are damaged, and they're cutting off the flow of oxygen to your heart. Your heart is choking to death because those vital arteries are clogged with plaque.

But before we get into a full discussion of how heart disease develops, let me define two important terms for you.

1. *Arteriosclerosis* is damage and hardening of the major arteries.

2. *Atherosclerosis* is fat and cholesterol buildup in the arteries.

These terms are sometimes used synonymously, even though they refer to two separate but related events—the two-step process of heart disease. First the arteries are damaged. Then plaque forms and creates blockages in the arteries. I will not use either of these terms, because they are technical and often confusing. But now, if you hear someone else use them, at least you'll know what they mean.

LIFE IS SHORT, ARTERIES ARE LONG

Placed end to end, all the blood vessels in the body would stretch some 60,000 miles in length. We are concerned here with roughly half of this mileage, the arteries.

Arteries are blood vessels that take oxygenated blood from the heart and distribute it throughout the body. The large arteries are muscular tubes lined with endothelial cells. These cells give the artery a smooth surface to facilitate blood flow and form a wall between the blood and the muscle cells of the artery walls. The endothelial cells also produce substances that thin the blood and prevent blood clots, dissolve small clots that do form, and prevent the underlying muscle cells from multiplying.

Like every other cell in the body, the muscle cells in arteries require a constant flow of oxygen. The outer layers of the artery wall have their own blood vessels. The inner layers have no blood vessels and depend on oxygen that is diffused from the blood carried by the arteries themselves through the endothelial cell wall.

Clumps of Fat

When there's too much fat in the blood, it causes the oxygen-carrying red blood cells to clump together. This disrupts the diffusion of oxygen, and the artery walls are literally starved for air. Without sufficient oxygen, the muscle cells are damaged and the artery walls swell. As the artery walls swell, the endothelial cells are stretched apart.

This experiment at home will serve as a visual example of the resulting damage to arterial walls: Take a balloon and blow it up halfway. Draw on it with a magic marker. Then blow it up the rest of the way. The ink from the magic marker will crack as the balloon expands, leaving gaps where there once was an unbroken line of color.

In the same way, endothelial cells spread apart, leaving areas of the artery walls unprotected. Left unprotected, the artery walls become damaged, allowing fat and cholesterol to enter the muscle layer of the artery. This is how plaque starts to form.

More Artery Enemies

High levels of fat aren't the only ways that artery walls can be damaged. Smoking is very bad for the arteries. It reduces oxygen in the blood by increasing carbon monoxide. And switching to a low-tar and low-nicotine cigarette won't help much. Any kind of smoking increases carbon monoxide and lowers the oxygen in your blood.

High blood pressure can also cause arterial damage, as the force of the circulating blood is increased, hurting the sensitive endothelial cells.

Cholesterol, which comes from animal fat, has been found not only to form blockages in the arteries, but to create the conditions in which these blockages begin. Studies have shown that even low concentrations of oxygenated cholesterol can cause severe arterial damage.

Low levels of vitamin C, moreover, seriously compromise artery walls. Since vitamin C is essential to the maintenance of the body's connective tissue, insufficient amounts of the nutrient may lead to weakening of the tissue bonding the endothelial cells. This makes it much easier for damage to occur.

SECOND STAGE OF HEART DISEASE

Once the arterial walls are damaged, the second stage of heart disease has a chance to develop.

If your blood cholesterol level is 150 or lower and your vitamin C levels are high, then whatever damage does occur to your arteries can be easily repaired. If your cholesterol is low, then plaque cannot easily form. Vitamin C both protects the artery linings and helps repair them once they are damaged. But if your cholesterol level is about average for an American (210) and you don't get enough vitamin C, your arteries are likely to get worse.

Cholesterol and fat leak through the endothelial damage and into the muscle layer of the artery. This irritates the muscle cells, and they begin to multiply, covering the cholesterol particles. The resulting buildup, as we have seen, is known as plaque. And if you don't lower your blood cholesterol levels, the plaque keeps accumulating, until the artery is blocked, or even completely closed.

HOW ARTERIES GET BLOCKED

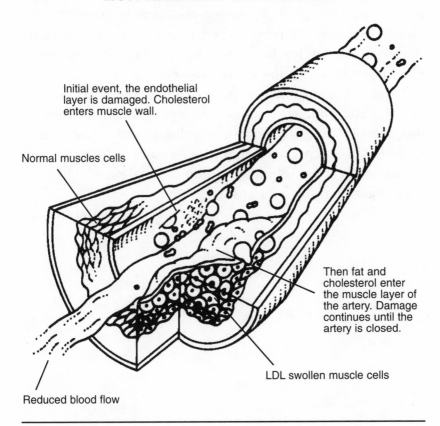

Initial event, the endothelial layer is damaged. Cholesterol enters muscle wall.

Normal muscles cells

Then fat and cholesterol enter the muscle layer of the artery. Damage continues until the artery is closed.

LDL swollen muscle cells

Reduced blood flow

HEART DISEASE, THE QUIET KILLER

Since there are no nerve endings inside your blood vessels, you cannot feel the effects of artery damage or plaque buildup. Your lifestyle could be killing you and you would not even know it.

Your coronary artery walls could be deteriorating right now, and you'd never feel a thing. Not until your heart started dying a little bit at a time.

Heart disease does not exhibit any symptoms until it has progressed enough to be dangerous, perhaps even deadly. One way to avoid the heart surgery trap is to ensure that heart disease won't develop in the first place. But to prevent heart disease you have to know its root causes.

There are many misconceptions concerning heart disease, and the conventional wisdom concerning this killer is often dangerously wrong. In the next few chapters I will discuss free radicals, cholesterol, and fat, the root causes of heart disease. Armed with correct information, you can make the right decisions regarding your own health.

CHAPTER NINE

Free Radicals: Where Heart Disease Begins

These little talked about byproducts of metabolism literally rust away the protective linings of our arteries.

Free radicals are the real culprit in heart disease. Yes, cholesterol, fat, inactivity, stress, and bad nutrition all play significant roles in clogging your coronary arteries. But the damage caused by free radicals is what allows them to do their dirty work.

Free radicals make heart disease possible. And curbing the damage they cause your arteries is the way to reverse heart disease and avoid the surgery trap.

A HOUSEHOLD PHRASE IN THE MAKING

You've never heard of free radicals? That's not surprising. Because even though the medical establishment has known about free radicals for years, somehow it has neglected to tell the public much about them.

I remember studying free radicals in medical school. But back then it was thought that free radicals concerned only physics and chemistry—not nutrition. Now we are beginning to discover that free radicals are the seeds of our bodies' own destruction.

Free radicals are the single most important discovery about health in some time. And while we already know their effect on the heart, free radicals could prove to be the link that scientists have needed to find cures for many other degenerative diseases, including ALS (Lou Gehrig's disease), Alzheimer's, arthritis, and even cancer.

Someday soon, "free radical damage" will be a household phrase.

SO WHAT ARE FREE RADICALS?

When you were a kid, did you ever leave your bicycle outside in the rain? It would quickly rust. And if you left the bike out long enough, it would become useless.

Well, our bodies break down in much the same way. Free radicals, like rust, are made by oxidation, which is a chemical change caused by exposure to oxygen. We think of oxygen as a good thing, and it generally is. But when it makes free radicals, it also creates the opportunity for significant damage. Your bike was perfectly safe sitting outside in the sunshine, but once it rained, and the water acted as a catalyst for oxidation, rust began to form. Rust is nothing more than oxygen-created free radicals, the same molecules that destroy our bodies, that make us grow old and get sick.

The Chemical Process

A free radical is thus named because it is an atom that has an unpaired electron, that is, an electrically charged particle spinning in lonely orbit and searching for another electron to counterbalance it. When free radicals come into contact with balanced molecules, they can either give their lonely particle away or steal an electron from the healthy molecule, causing significant damage.

A free radical is desperate to hook up with another molecule that will cure its missing electron problem. It will latch onto whatever molecule is available. Free radicals are extremely toxic to cell membranes, proteins, and even the DNA of your chromosomes. When free radicals attack the DNA, they cause mutations that could result in cancer. When they attack skin cells, pulling electrons out of healthy cells, they make wrinkles.

As damage builds up, cells get sick. Some of them die. The cells that do not reproduce themselves, like muscle, brain, and eye cells, are particularly vulnerable. This is why, as we age, we get weak, have memory loss, and develop cataracts.

If free radicals are not contained, they will corrode everything they touch. And they can start a chain reaction by producing other free radicals, until the damage they do spreads out of control, like a brush fire that has started from the flame of a single match.

The most common and dangerous free radicals are those created by oxygen. Just like the oxidized rust that formed on your bike, these free radicals do incredible injury to our bodies by deforming or corroding every molecule they come into contact with.

WHY DOES THE BODY CREATE FREE RADICALS?

Ironically, the seeds of our demise are the byproducts of life. We must have energy, and we obtain energy by burning foodstuffs, a process for which oxygen is necessary. Free radicals are the byproducts of vital activity. They are continually generated by the body in the digestion of food, production of energy, detoxification of poisons, and in fighting off pathogens.

Our bodies' wide array of enzymes and antioxidant nutrients helps rein free radicals in, stopping them from doing extensive damage. If enough antioxidants and enzymes are available, free radicals are deactivated.

As long as they're produced internally and naturally, free radicals are simply the inevitable fallout from life. But when you introduce more free radicals than your body can handle, or let your antioxidant free radical defenses down, then you're in trouble.

FREE RADICALS AND HEART DISEASE

Free radicals are the primary cause of plaque buildup in the arteries. Without free radical damage the arteries would remain smooth, and fat and cholesterol, having nowhere to latch onto, would be unable to accumulate. Unfortunately, free radicals compromise the arterial walls and allow plaque to attach to them.

Think of your arteries as a system of pipes. Very delicate, very complicated pipes, but pipes nonetheless. As long as your pipes are clean, all the gunk that is traveling through them will get where it needs to go without leaving much residue. But if your pipes are rusty, and there's a lot of gunk passing through, some of it will get stuck on the rough surface of the pipes. Then more gunk starts attaching itself to the gunk that's already built up. And pretty soon you've got clogged pipes.

How do free radicals rust your arteries?

A free radical with an unpaired electron is spinning around, seeking another molecule to steal from to bring it back into balance. If it's in the area of a coronary artery and it finds a lipid, or fat, molecule, it will yank a positively charged proton off. The lipid is now missing a proton, which it in turn steals from its neighbor. This causes a chain reaction, which eventually causes damage to the membrane itself.

The disruption to normal cells caused by this one free radical has created an ideal environment for plaque formation. But that's not all that free radicals do to advance heart disease. They can also block the production of the hormone prostaglandin, causing spasms and blood clots in the arteries. And they can interact with fats in particularly ugly ways.

FREE RADICALS AND FATS

One reason a high-fat diet is so unhealthy is that it increases the amount of free radicals in the body. A lower fat diet calms the free-radical storm.

Countless studies have linked heart disease with increased intakes of fat. Now we know why. High-fat levels create high free-radical levels, and the free radicals deteriorate the artery walls at a rapid rate. In turn, high-fat levels create more cholesterol to form plaque on the damaged artery walls. Because of their double-barreled attack on arteries, lipid peroxides— the free radicals formed from fat—are our main concern in cardiovascular health.

Cholesterol, fats, and particularly unsaturated fats are routinely "radicalized" by oxygen into lipid peroxides. The free radical that attacked and destroyed the cell membrane described above was a fat (lipid) peroxide. In much the same way that oxygen eats away at the metal parts of that bicycle you left out in the rain, oxygen eats away at fats, which then become free radicals and begin eating away at the cell linings of your arteries. To avoid heart disease you have to limit your intake of fat and thus reduce free-radical activity.

Oxidation, which occurs whenever fats are exposed to oxygen, is the reason food goes rancid. If you have ever bitten into a rancid nut, you've gotten a mouth full of free radicals. They're not too tasty, are they? Also, the more any food is prepared, processed, or in any way altered from its original, whole form, the more free radicals it contains; and the more these free radicals will damage your body when you ingest them. Heat is also a powerful catalyst for oxidation, so the less you cook foods, especially fatty foods, the fewer free radicals you will be introducing into your body.

In addition to oxidation, lipid peroxides are created inside the body by the ionizing radiation of X rays and sources of electromagnetic radiation, like that produced by television and computer screens. So many of the "conveniences" of modern life, such as fast food and computers, are also free-radical factories.

NOW THE GOOD NEWS

Since free radicals are produced by the very systems that are essential to life, the body has an elaborate system to defend against them. The key players on this defense team are called antioxidants—vitamin C, vitamin E, vitamin A, beta carotene, selenium, copper, zinc, manganese, and certain sulphur-containing amino acids such as L-cysteine.

Some of the protectors are intracellular (inside the cell), mopping up free radicals produced by the metabolism, while others are extracellular (outside the cell), protecting the lining of the artery wall from free radicals flowing in the blood. This defense system has to be strong in every way, because free radicals will exploit any weakness, and inside the body the stakes are high.

TRIPLE PROTECTION

Antioxidants protect the body from free radicals in three ways:

Antioxidants prevent free-radical production. Try this experiment at home: Crush a 500 mg tablet of vitamin C, or use the crystalline form. Next, cut an apple in half and immediately spread a thin coat of the powdered vitamin C on the cut side of one half. Leave the other half alone. Let both halves sit side by side, and in just a few minutes you will see that the unprotected half turns brown as it reacts with oxygen in the air, while the half protected by vitamin C remains white and fresh.

Antioxidants have the same effect inside your body. A good amount of antioxidant nutrients will limit the production of free radicals much in the same way that they protect an apple from turning brown.

Antioxidants put out the brush fire before it spreads. They interrupt the damaging chain reaction started by free radicals. This is particularly important when the free radicals attack the lipid layer of the cell membrane. Since lipid molecules are so concentrated in the membrane, the entire cell would be destroyed were it not for antioxidants, particularly vitamin E.

Antioxidants neutralize free-radical particles before they have a chance to do damage. For instance, beta carotene is particularly good at neutralizing singlet oxygen, a reactive particle capable of generating and being transformed into more toxic free radicals. Beta carotene does this by absorbing the destructive energy of singlet oxygen into its own molecular structure and slowly discharging this energy in a safe manner.

Each element of the body's anti-free-radical defense system helps by itself to protect the body, but the system depends on

---------- **FREE-RADICAL CATALYSTS** ----------

These substances act as catalysts for free radicals, and you should limit your exposure to them as much as possible.

Aluminum—cans, foil, antacids, pots and pans, baking powder, deodorants, tap water, many drugs

Cadmium—batteries, cigarette smoke, coffee, gasoline, metal pipes

Carbon Monoxide—auto exhaust, cigarette smoke, smog

Chlorine—tap water, pools, the breakdown of table salt

Copper—excessive tap water, plumbing

Fluoride—tap water, toothpastes, dental work

Hexavalent Chromium—smog, tap water, cigarette smoke

Lead—dyes, gasoline, paint, plumbing, auto exhaust

Mercury—amalgam fillings, fish, film, paint, some cosmetics

Nitrates and Nitrites—processed meats, tap water

Polynuclear Aromatic Hydrocarbons—almost anything that burns

Synthetic Drugs—antibiotics, painkillers, barbiturates, illegal drugs

---

the interaction among these ingredients. So you have to make sure you get enough of all your antioxidants. Vitamin E has been shown to be much more effective in the presence of vitamin C. L-Cysteine is necessary for the production of glutathione, which requires adequate amounts of selenium. And glutathione is one of the most important antioxidants inside the cell.

Also, without proper nutrition, your body won't be able to make the enzymes that control free radicals. In the absence of these all-important enzymes, free radicals roam around unchecked doing grave damage to your heart and to your entire body.

Later I will go into more detail about what to do about free radicals in your body. For now, all you really need to know is that fighting back against free radicals (rather than having your chest ripped open by a surgeon) should be your first line of defense against heart disease.

WHAT ELSE CAN I DO ABOUT FREE RADICALS?

First of all, stop swallowing them. Eating a breakfast of scrambled eggs dished from a heated container, fried sausage or bacon loaded with oxidized fat and "radicalized" nitrosamines, and hash browns deep fried in superheated oils (probably the most dangerous supplier of free radicals) is like throwing a bucket of hot coals into a hay barn. Deep fried foods are definitely out. But cut down your intake of "lightly sauteed" ones as well.

Every day eat a large salad and one or two carrots. These are natural sources of free-radical scavengers, particularly beta carotene, vitamin C, and other nutritional elements that we don't know about and certainly haven't put in capsules.

The ideal situation is to achieve a balance between free radicals and antioxidants. The closer you come to that balance, the better off you are.

RUSTOLEUM FOR YOUR ARTERIES

Remember that old bike you left out in the rain? The parts that rusted, like the gear spokes and the chain, were exposed metal. But the frame and the wheels, which were protected by paint and chrome, didn't rust. In the same way your bike is protected by paint and chrome, you can minimize the damage that free radicals do to your arteries. By eating a good, healthy diet and taking antioxidant supplements, you can protect yourself against free-radical damage and stop heart disease before it gets a chance to start. It's easier, more effective, and a whole lot safer than bypass surgery.

CHAPTER TEN

The Cholesterol Controversy

Killer cholesterol, lifesaving cholesterol, and how to reduce the first and raise the second.

Unless you've been living in a cave for the past twenty years, you know that cholesterol can kill you. But did you also know that without cholesterol you would die?

That does not mean you should eat a dozen eggs for breakfast. The body manufactures all the cholesterol it needs. In fact, the body produces the same amount of cholesterol no matter how much is ingested, so the cholesterol you eat is simply added to the amount the body makes. Even if you cut all cholesterol out of your diet, your body would make sure you had enough. And since cholesterol itself has no nutritive value, there's no need to eat it at all. Nor would we except that we live in a culture that promotes the eating of animal protein. And that diet is literally killing us.

A KILLER AMONG US

For almost forty years, most authorities have agreed that an elevated blood cholesterol level is associated with an increased risk of heart disease and heart attack. And the higher the blood cholesterol level, the greater the risk.

Good Cholesterol, Bad Cholesterol

If these are the facts, why the controversy? To understand that, we need to understand just what cholesterol is and how it moves through the body.

Cholesterol is a versatile compound that serves three main functions in humans. It is used to manufacture steroids or cortisonelike hormones, including sex hormones; it helps the liver produce bile; and it is a main component of cell membranes and structures, a kind of building block for body tissues. Without cholesterol, we would literally fall apart.

The problem arises when the body has too much cholesterol. The excess is deposited inside the walls of the coronary arteries, creating a lack of oxygen to the heart muscle. It can also form in other arteries, including those feeding the brain, which could cause a stroke.

Since cholesterol is a fatty substance, it cannot mix with the blood, which is water based. To travel through the body, it must be packaged into special molecules called lipoproteins. The fatty cholesterol is wrapped inside a water-soluble protein coating that allows it to flow through the blood.

These lipoproteins move cholesterol through the body, taking it to tissues that need it and removing it from areas that don't. The main lipoproteins carrying cholesterol around the body are called low-density lipoproteins, or LDL cholesterol. You may have heard of LDL referred to as the "bad" cholesterol because it is the mechanism by which cholesterol is deposited in the arteries.

HDL cholesterol (high-density lipoprotein) is known as the "good" cholesterol because it helps remove cholesterol from the blood and eventually transports it to the liver for excretion.

Another form of cholesterol is VLDL (very low density lipoprotein) which is manufactured by the liver as a precursor for LDL cholesterol production. VLDL also transports triglycerides, blood fats produced by the liver.

Beyond "Good" and "Bad"

For almost two decades, LDL cholesterol has been the undisputed troublemaker because it transports cholesterol throughout the body. And for just about as long, HDL has been the undisputed do-gooder because it gets rid of cholesterol. But recent information has cast new light on the HDL particle. We now know that HDL comes in two types, one good and the other not so good.

We've long known that LDL and HDL particles have cholesterol and phospholipids inside and protein strands wrapped around the outside. Recent findings show that HDL particles may have one of two protein wrappers, technically known as A-I and A-II.

Dr. H. Bryan Brewer of the Molecular Disease Laboratory at the National Heart, Blood, and Lung Institute in Rockville, Maryland, discovered that we benefit only from the A-I HDL particle, not from the A-II type.

HDL levels are considered dangerously low at 35 milligrams or lower, yet Dr. Brewer reported on a seventy-year-old woman who had an HDL level as low as 7 milligrams. She had no heart disease. An examination showed her HDL was almost entirely of the A-I type. Even though her levels were low, the A-I type protected her.

Dr. Brewer also reported on a middle-aged man who had an HDL level of 8 milligrams. An examination of his HDL showed that it was almost entirely type A-II; he had a heart attack at age forty-two.

Researchers are still learning about the two HDL types. But what has been proven so far is that the dichotomy of "good" and "bad" cholesterol is not as simple as it originally seemed.

The Protein Flag

Another aspect of cholesterol research that has not received the attention it deserves concerns the relationship between cholesterol and vitamin C.

Low-density lipoprotein(a) is an offshoot of the LDL ("bad") cholesterol particle, with a small strand of protein attached to the outside that looks like a flag. This protein flag makes the lipoprotein(a) particles sticky, which allows them to adhere to and protect damaged or cut arterial walls.

Dr. Matthias Rath, a German researcher, discovered that these particles quickly build up into arterial plaque. Dr. Linus Pauling, building on Rath's discovery, found high levels of lipoprotein(a) in the bloodstream only of mammals who no longer produced vitamin C.[1]

The doctors found that the two substances had a directly inverse relationship in the body. Lipoprotein(a) levels shot up when vitamin C levels were low and decreased when vitamin C levels were high. They also showed that very low levels of vitamin C could cause arterial atherosclerotic disease in guinea pigs and that the disease could be reversed by boosting the vitamin C level.

The protein flag, the two physicians concluded, by its ability to adhere to damaged arterial walls, was designed to protect mammals who could no longer produce beneficial vitamin C.[2]

Without Vitamin C, which enables tissue to heal properly, lipoprotein(a) steps in and acts as a bandage. The problem, however, is that when vitamin C levels are low, lipoprotein(a) begins to build up on artery walls and thickens into plaque, making the cholesterol particle dangerous. Obviously, vitamin C levels should be kept reasonably high.

WHAT'S THE AVERAGE?

Some laboratories issue a graph in which the normal range for blood cholesterol is between 150 and 300. That's like saying a safe rate of driving speed is between 55 and 155 mph. The average American's blood cholesterol level is about 210, which is dangerously close to the average level of heart patients (about 220). Dr. Robert Wissler, of the University of Chicago, and Dr. William Castelli, who directed a series of studies of cholesterol, show that a cholesterol level of 150 or lower nearly guarantees immunity from heart disease.

As your total blood cholesterol level increases, so does your risk. A person with a level of 190 has a measurable risk of heart attack, but a person with a level of 260 has a risk five times as great.

One of the effects of our high cholesterol levels is that we tend to think of the condition as being normal. But just because a cholesterol level of 210 is in the median range doesn't mean it's healthy. It just means that there are a lot of people who are sicker than average. Doctors commonly give their patients a false sense of security by telling them that their blood cholesterol level is normal when in fact it is dangerously high. Perhaps that helps explain why so many heart attacks come without warning. If only these people knew how sick their hearts were, perhaps they would have done something about it before it was too late.

SOURCES OF CHOLESTEROL

All foods that come from animals contain some form of cholesterol. There is no cholesterol in any vegetable or grain. Even low-fat animal foods like chicken or fish contain cholesterol, while high-vegetable-fat foods like peanut butter and margarine have no cholesterol.

Animal foods can be broken down into three separate groups. Some of these foods may be low in fat, but still have high cholesterol.

- *Group 1: Flesh foods that consist of fish, chicken, and meat.* They contain about 20 to 25 mg of cholesterol per ounce.

- *Group 2: Organ meats, like liver, kidneys, and brain.* These contain the highest concentration of cholesterol, from 70 to 120 mg per ounce.

- *Group 3: Eggs.* One single egg contains 215 mg of cholesterol. Eggs are the single major source of cholesterol in the average American's diet, and contribute from 30 to 55 percent of all cholesterol intake.

But skipping the omelet won't make you safe.

Remember that a lot of other foods contain eggs. Baked goods like muffins and danishes, breads and cakes, pancakes and waffles, even pastas can have significant cholesterol levels. On the other hand, all of the egg's cholesterol is in the yolk, so an egg white omelet or rice pudding made with skim milk and egg whites can be a healthy alternative to their high-fat, high-cholesterol counterparts.

ORIENTAL VS. WESTERN DIETS

Studies comparing Japanese and other Oriental diets with American diets reveal an interesting fact. Eastern diets are built around rices and fruits that are high in carbohydrates, not in saturated fat foods and animal proteins. And when a culture's diet is low in fat, it has a low rate of heart disease. Studies have shown that when Japanese migrate to Western countries and adopt our diet and lifestyle, they adopt our heart disease levels too—in the course of just one generation. It's chilling to think how quickly our diets can destroy us.

Clear and convincing evidence in both human and animal studies shows that a lower fat, higher complex carbohydrate diet without saturated fats or cholesterol actually reverses the cholesterol buildup on artery walls and decreases the risk of heart disease.

THE SATURATION MYTH

Beyond blood cholesterol concentration, a high-cholesterol diet holds another risk—cholesterol saturation. The body can only assimilate so much cholesterol a day. If you take in any more, it simply passes through the colon. And that, according to many studies, represents a significant cancer risk. Cholesterol saturation (not to be confused with saturated fats) can be reached at levels of 600 to 750 mg of cholesterol a day, which is a typical American diet.

A misperception has been created by the saturation factor. Several studies have appeared in the past few years that have been misinterpreted in the popular press as having proved that animal cholesterol intake had little or no impact on blood cholesterol levels. Since many Americans are consuming cholesterol at saturation levels, tests giving them even more cholesterol may not result in higher levels of blood cholesterol. So, when someone tells you that it doesn't matter what you eat, since your cholesterol level will stay the same, tell them that they're wrong.

FREE RADICAL CHOLESTEROL

The final overlooked piece about cholesterol is this: Heat and oxygen dangerously alter LDL cholesterol.

When exposed to those elements, LDL becomes infested with free radicals, the destructive atoms that roam around in your body spoiling healthy cells. In fact, free radicals oxidize cholesterol into more than four hundred toxic substances.

This makes some cholesterols far more dangerous than others. The cholesterol in stored powdered eggs, for example, suffers from overexposure to oxygen. Exposure to intense heat means deep fried foods and baked goods are much worse than fresh or lightly cooked foods.

Eat fresh foods and cook lightly. Make it as tough as you can for free radicals to get a toehold.

AND THE BAND PLAYED ON

That doctors know about the health hazards of cholesterol doesn't mean they are prepared to do anything about it. God forbid they tell their patients how to live their lives. Besides, many of these doctors are probably eating high levels of animal cholesterol themselves, even though they know better.

Everybody knows that there is a connection between diet and blood cholesterol. Everybody knows that there is a connection between cholesterol and heart disease. Everyone knows that heart disease is a killer. Why then are so few willing to do anything about it? Because the animal protein diet is such a strong part of our culture (and economy) that the social cost of 500,000 deaths a year seems to be a small price to pay for the right to have our eggs for breakfast, hamburgers for lunch, and steaks for dinner.

CHAPTER ELEVEN

The Truth About Fats

How a high fat diet suffocates your cells.
The only two fats you'll ever need.

Fat clogs your arteries and thickens your blood, transforming your once vigorous circulatory system into a sclerotic transmitter of deadly sludge. Without fat, heart attacks wouldn't happen.

Think of free radicals, cholesterol, and fat as three bad guys who walk into a peaceful frontier town and start shooting up the place. Although they each have specific roles, they always work as a team. And you can't get rid of just one of them, you've got to take out all three.

STRANGLED BY FAT

Try holding your breath. You're okay for a few seconds. Then your head starts to pound. You feel strangled. Your lungs ache. You start feeling weak, a little dizzy. Your body is panicking. It needs oxygen.

Now breathe deeply. Doesn't that feel much better? Doesn't it make much more sense?

You certainly wouldn't go through your day holding your breath. Then why are you eating fatty foods? Fat in your diet works much the same way, limiting the supply of oxygen to the body, and virtually strangling you.

RIVERS OF OXYGEN

You need oxygen, lots of it, all the time. Every one of the millions of cells that make up your body requires a constantly replenished supply of it. Without enough oxygen, your body just doesn't work right. If the supply of oxygen is completely cut off, you will die.

Oxygen is carried through the bloodstream by red blood cells. They pick up oxygen in the lungs and travel to the heart, where they are pumped to other parts of the body. To reach the cells that need oxygen nourishment, they must go through the capillaries, the smallest blood vessels in your body. The capillaries are only about five microns in diameter (a micron is one ten-thousandth of a centimer) and red blood cells are about seven microns in size—larger than the path they must follow. This sounds like a problem. But in fact, that's the way nature planned it. You see, it's the job of the capillaries to get the oxygen from the red blood cells so it can pass the nourishment on to the surrounding tissues. And by being slightly larger than their path, the red blood cells must squeeze through single file, coming right up against the cells to which they then transfer their oxygen. Having delivered their load of oxygen, they pick up carbon dioxide and other waste products for disposal.

At least that's the way your body is supposed to work. But when you eat a meal that's loaded with fat, you mess up the whole system.

DAMMING THE RIVER

Ever try to wash a greasy frying pan? Plain old hot water won't do it. Instead you have to use soap, usually some liquid detergent that's specially designed to fight grease. And even that can leave a slimy film on the pan, because fat isn't water soluble. It just doesn't dissolve.

The same thing happens in your body. While other food components are broken down and metabolized, the body can't digest fat. Instead it is emulsified into little droplets called "chylomicrons." And rather than traveling to the liver, for processing and delivery throughout the body, fat is processed by the lymphatic system, which dumps the fat directly into the blood stream. The heart then has to pump all this unprocessed sludge into the blood vessels.

So, while your blood is trying to deliver fresh oxygen and nutrients to the cells of the body, there's all this fat in the way. It's as if you're trying to deliver a very important package across town and you're stuck in a traffic jam created by a bunch of Sunday drivers.

Not only does fat get in the way but, in the same way that grease sticks to your frying pan, fat coats the red blood cells and makes them stick together. These clumps of red blood cells are now too large to get through the capillaries. And your body can't get the oxygen it needs, or dispose of the wastes it has accumulated.

———— FAT BLOCKS OXYGEN DELIVERY ————

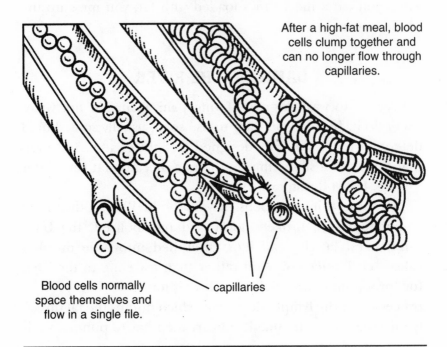

After a high-fat meal, blood cells clump together and can no longer flow through capillaries.

Blood cells normally space themselves and flow in a single file.

capillaries

FAT AND ANGINA

Your heart gets its oxygen the same way as all the other parts of the body, through capillaries. So if your red blood cells can't pass through the capillaries, you are cutting off oxygen to the heart.

What happens when oxygen to the heart is diminished? Angina, or sharp, shooting pains in the chest, occur. Every attack of angina is a cry from the heart for more oxygen. And it is often the warning sign of heart disease and a possible heart attack.

Studies have shown that even one high-fat meal can greatly impede the supply of oxygen to the heart and bring on angina. So, the next time you have a craving for a big, greasy bacon cheeseburger with a side of fries and a chocolate milkshake, remember that eating that much fat is like holding your breath for a very, very long time.

IS THAT A GOOD FAT OR A BAD FAT?

All fats are bad for you when taken in excess. But you need a certain amount of fat in your diet. And some fats are actually good for you, in moderation.

If you are on a low- or non-fat diet, you may be neglecting essential fats and oils. But if you are on a typically high-fat American diet, you could be killing yourself.

So, how can you tell a good fat from a bad fat?

Essential Fats: Linolenic and Linoleic Acids

There are two good fats. Both of them are essential fatty acids, which means that they are necessary for normal cell structure and body function. (All fats are fatty acids, which means they are one part fatty, which is not water soluble, and one part acid, which is.) One is alpha-linolenic acid (LNA), an omega-3 fatty acid, and the other is linoleic acid (LA), an omega-6 fatty acid.

Our bodies cannot produce these essential fatty acids; you must get them from your diet.

If you can get both omega-3 fatty acids and omega-6 fatty acids into your diet, you've satisfied your need for fats because all other fats can be manufactured from these. You don't need any other fats.

Both LNA and LA fatty acids function as components of nerve cells, cell membranes, and hormonelike substances known as prostaglandins. But they also have some significant differences that are proving to be quite valuable to researchers. Scientists are discovering that by manipulating the levels of dietary oils, body function can be altered dramatically. Omega-3 oils can reduce cholesterol, relieve angina, bring down high blood pressure, and help arthritis, psoriasis, and eczema.

But in addition to their possible curative powers, it is always necessary to maintain a proper level of essential fats. When you've got the right fats in your diet, the benefits are innumerable: smooth skin; clear arteries; optimum brain, hormonal, and biochemical function and reactions; a stimulated metabolism; and a trim body because of an increased burning rate of fats and glucose.

Likewise, a deficiency of these essential fatty acids leads to a host of health problems and is associated with heart disease, cancer, diabetes, and various other degenerative illnesses.[1]

Not surprisingly, the level of essential fatty acids is significantly lower in heart attack patients than in other people.

Getting Enough Good Fats If you are eating a primarily vegetarian diet, with an ample amount of fresh foods, particularly deep-green leafy vegetables that are high in linolenic acid, as well as a variety of fresh nuts and seeds that can be used as snack foods, you are getting an ample supply of essential fatty acids.

The problem with our modern diet is that many of the oils we use, particularly in cooking, are significantly altered by heat and processing, which converts good unsaturated fats into not-so-good saturated fats. On top of that, we eat a substantial amount of animal fat, which simply adds calories and elevates cholesterol levels.

Fats to Avoid

You've probably heard it before—a food product claims to be low in saturated fat. Or your doctor tell you to stick to unsaturated fat. What do these terms mean?

Basically, unsaturated fats are better for you than saturated fats. But as we have seen before with "good" and "bad" cholesterol, that distinction is not as significant as some people would have you think.

Unsaturated Fats Monounsaturated fats like canola, olive, peanut, and cashew oil are liquid at room temperature, but may become solid in the refrigerator. Foods high in monounsaturated fats include avocados, cashews, olives, and peanuts. Polyunsaturated fats like cottonseed, safflower, sunflower, and soybean oils are liquid even in cold temperatures. Foods high in polyunsaturated fats include almonds, fish, margarine, mayonnaise, pecans, and walnuts.

Since doctors have been recommending unsaturated fats as being healthier than saturated ones, the American diet now contains unprecedented amounts of unsaturated fat. That may be better than the same levels of saturated fats, but not by much. Unsaturated fats still create fat and cholesterol in the bloodstream. And studies have found a connection between polyunsaturates and cancer, immune system repression, and gallstones.

Saturated Fats Saturated fats are just plain bad. They offer no nutritive benefits and create a whole host of health problems. You'd think that sensible people would stay away from a food that did them no good and a great deal of harm. Unfortunately, the American diet is still loaded with saturated fats.

About the only thing saturated fats do is give us energy. But there are much better ways to get energy, like complex carbohydrates. Saturated fats also produce bile. Since bile absorbs fat, that should be good for us, right? Actually, not. Bile is good only when our diets are fiber-rich, and most American diets aren't. Without fiber, the bile sits around in the intestinal tract and generates toxic substances, which are eventually excreted.

In addition to helping create cholesterol, saturated fat interferes with the removal of cholesterol from the blood and actually raises cholesterol levels. So, if you eat a cholesterol-free food that has a lot of saturated fats, you are still increasing your risk of heart disease.

Want to hear more? Saturated fats weaken cell membranes, allowing viruses, bacteria, and fungi to get inside. They weaken the immune system. And they make you fat.

Saturated fats can be found in most animal foods, such as meat, eggs, milk, and cheese. They are also in tropical oils, like coconut oil, palm oil, and cocoa butter. They tend to be solid at room temperature.

Stay away from saturated fats.

Triglycerides: Good Fats Gone Bad   Once in the body, fats like to bond with proteins or glycerol molecules to form lipoproteins and triglycerides, respectively. We talked about lipoproteins in the cholesterol chapter, but triglycerides are a new subject for us.

High levels of triglycerides in the blood indicate that a diet is heavy in nonessential fatty acids and refined carbohydrates. Unfortunately, when triglycerides break down in our bodies during various chemical interactions, they break back into the unhealthy nonessential fats.

Triglycerides play a major role in maintaining the effectiveness of our cell membranes. So, when triglycerides have lots of saturated fats in them, cell membranes become hard and inflexible. Consequently, the cell's ability to function freely is reduced.

These fats can also cause clotting because they thicken the blood cells and make them too big to travel through the tiniest capillaries.

Indecent Exposure   Air, heat, radiation, and light can alter the chemical makeup of a fat in the blink of an eye, turning it into an agent of heart disease.

We generally think of oxygen as a positive thing, but fats tend not to like it much. Antioxidants, whether nutrients or supplements, counteract oxidation more or less by diverting the oxygen atom so it won't bond with the unsaturated fatty acid. Antioxidants give the oxygen an atom to bond with so it leaves the fatty acid alone. That's how vitamins C, E, and B; selenium; and beta carotene protect you.

Even if you're taking antioxidants, you want to stay away from oxidized fats. High heat quickly oxidizes unsaturated fatty acids and makes them unhealthy. Baking is no different. It is the heat, not the method of applying it, that produces the oxidation.

Unfortunately, this is true even of Chinese and other Oriental cooking. Health-conscious people who choose Oriental restaurants for their rice and vegetables should be aware that heating the oil to high temperatures, while constantly exposing it to light and air, eliminates many of the low-fat benefits of Oriental cuisine.

Native Orientals stir fry using crude, not highly processed, oil. And they put water in the wok first to keep the oil temperature down, greatly reducing the potential for an unhealthy conversion. They also eat a lot of fiber and high-nutrient foods that help keep their heart disease rates down.

Though cooking oils are an integrated part of American life, it is wisest to steer away from them and develop a taste for foods that have not been fried or sautéed in hot oils.

How Much Fat?

I recommend that your fat intake not exceed 15 to 20 percent of your total caloric intake. Thus, a person who consumes 1,800 calories daily can consume 360 of those calories in fat, which is about 40 grams of fat, or the equivalent of about 2 1/2 tablespoons of oil.

Get your essential fatty acids from fresh vegetables. For the omega-3 fatty acids, supplement the vegetable intake with capsules of fish oil, or 1 to 2 tablespoons of flax seed oil as a food supplement.

Cutting Fat Is Not Enough

Reducing fat is an important step in reversing heart disease. But you have to be careful that you are still getting your essential fatty acids. And it won't do to simply go on a low- or nonfat diet, if other needed lifestyle changes don't go along with it. We'll discuss these necessary changes in later chapters.

CHAPTER TWELVE

What About Blood Pressure?

**Why it matters, how to reduce it, and why
beta blockers and other new "miracle drugs"
may be wrong for you.**

If you are curious about what high blood pressure is like inside your arteries, just cover the spout of a running garden hose with your thumb. All of a sudden enough water backs up to make the hose go stiff and the water starts squirting out. If you really stop up the opening, you can cause a rupture in the hose—a seam will break and water will leak out all over.

That's exactly what's going on in your circulatory system when you've got high blood pressure.

Of course, you need some blood pressure, otherwise your blood wouldn't circulate. But high blood pressure is dangerous, especially if you have fatty buildup in the arteries. High blood pressure speeds up the hardening of arteries caused by free radicals and fat. The increased pressure on the inner walls of the arteries makes them much more vulnerable to a buildup of fatty deposits. Also, clots could form in arteries that have already been narrowed by plaque formation. A clot in a coronary artery can result in a heart attack. One clot in an artery in your neck, or in a blood vessel in your brain, can cause a stroke.

High blood pressure also causes the heart to work harder, which means it needs more oxygen. With this extra work load, the heart could become stiff and weak, unable to pump blood efficiently.

WHAT DO THOSE NUMBERS MEAN?

When you go to the doctor and he takes your blood pressure, the result is read in two different numbers. The first number is the systolic or contraction reading. That's the pressure in your arteries when your heart is pumping. The second number is the diastolic or expanding pressure. That's the measurement when your heart is resting between beats.

As both systolic and diastolic readings rise, your chance of heart disease, congestive heart failure, stroke, or kidney disease increases. That's the bad news. The good news is that high blood pressure is treatable and reversible.

NOT A DISEASE

High blood pressure is not a disease; it's a condition.

Some forms of high blood pressure are unavoidable, but for most it's the price paid for living and eating the way we do. High blood pressure is a common chronic condition, affecting up to 60 million people in the United States alone. It is the leading cause of strokes and a major risk factor in heart attacks.

CAUSES OF HIGH BLOOD PRESSURE

Many factors contribute to high blood pressure, and almost all of them are controllable:

High salt intake—not just table salt, but also the sodium that is found in much processed food.

High sugar intake—especially when these sugars are taken in simple form, rather than in complex carbohydrates.

Fat imbalance—too much saturated fat and not enough of the essential fatty acids to clear the system of fat solids.

Lack of nutrients—a diet low in vitamins and minerals, specifically potassium, calcium, magnesium, and vitamin C.

Lifestyle conditions—smoking, alcohol, too much caffeine, lack of exercise, and stress.

THE DRUG PROBLEM

Tens of millions of people are taking some kind of medication to lower their blood pressure. Many of them should leave those drugs alone.

Sometimes drugs are justified, but in many cases prescription synthetic drugs can be more dangerous to your health than the high blood pressure that they are trying to cure.

There are two kinds of high-blood-pressure drugs. Diuretics, commonly called water pills, lower blood pressure by increasing the kidney's excretion of sodium, which in turn reduces the volume of blood. The less blood your heart is pumping through your arteries, the lower your blood pressure. That may sound like a dandy cure, but it isn't.

The problem with diuretics is that they deplete your supplies of potassium and magnesium while at the same time elevating your triglyceride and cholesterol levels. These effects increase your risk of a heart attack and cardiac arrhythmias (irregular heartbeats). They increase the consistency of the blood, raise uric acid levels, and increase the stickiness of the platelets, which makes them more likely to form clots. Indeed, studies have shown that vigorous treatment with these drugs can actually increase the death rate.

The other common blood pressure drug, beta blockers, lower blood pressure by working through the nervous system. They block responses from beta nerve receptors, resulting in a slower heart rate and reducing the amount of blood that the heart pumps each minute. Beta blockers are notorious for causing impotence, fatigue, and depression. They also raise triglyceride and cholesterol levels. By reducing heart function, they make it difficult to get enough blood to the hands, feet, and brain, which is what accounts for many of the side effects. Long-term use of these drugs can lead to heart failure.

More recent entries to the high blood pressure drug sweepstakes are calcium channel blockers. They block the passage of calcium into the muscle cells that control the size of blood vessels. Since all muscles need calcium to constrict, when the muscles of the arteries are prevented from constricting, blood vessels dilate, allowing blood to flow more easily through them.

Calcium channel blockers also weaken the heart and can damage the liver. Magnesium, the natural calcium channel blocker, essentially does the same thing as these drugs without side effects.

The pharmaceutical cornucopia of drugs is incomprehensible to me, because the overwhelming majority of high-blood-pressure cases can be treated with diet and other lifestyle changes.

THREE SAFE STEPS TO LOWER
HIGH BLOOD PRESSURE

➤ *Go on a low fat diet.* Fat should comprise no more than 15 percent of your total daily intake of calories. Fat elevates blood pressure by increasing the thickness of the blood and stimulating hormones that cause the blood vessels to constrict. Reducing the fat in your diet will also stimulate weight loss, which almost always lowers blood pressure.

➤ *Increase magnesium and potassium.* You should take 1,000 mg per day of elemental magnesium. This supplement, along with two or three servings a day of fresh fruits and deep-green leafy vegetables (parsley, romaine lettuce, kale, broccoli), is what you need to achieve the therapeutic benefits of magnesium.

Surely you have heard that salt elevates blood pressure, but that is only half the story. Inadequate intake of potassium is the other. In general, when your sodium: potassium ratio is kept low, your blood pressure will drop. You can achieve this by eating more potassium-containing and less sodium-packed foods. Potassium is so rich and readily available in foods that you don't need to take supplements to get an optimal supply. Sources of potassium include tangerines, oranges, bananas, dried peas, and beans.

➤ *Exercise.* You should be exercising at least twenty minutes a day, three days a week. This will help lower your blood pressure by relaxing the muscles of your blood vessel walls and allowing them to expand, and by decreasing the thickness of your blood. Induced sweating also purges your body of excess sodium.

FOR QUICK RESULTS

The program above should produce results in about three to six weeks. But if you need to lower your blood pressure fast, and if you can muster the discipline, I suggest going on a rice and fruit diet. This was popularized by Walter Kempner in the 1940s. He found that severely hypertensive patients taking very powerful drugs would "depressurize" very rapidly by sticking to rice and fruit, which are low in fat and sodium, and high in potassium and magnesium.[1]

One day an airline pilot came to my clinic with blood pressure of 225/115 and announced, "If I don't have normal blood pressure in two weeks, I'll lose my license." I put him on a rice, fruit, and vegetable diet. Two weeks later he passed his flight physical with blood pressure of 130/84.

PART THREE

The Whitaker Wellness Program

CHAPTER THIRTEEN

Getting Well With the Four Pillars of Therapy

How thousands of patients have reversed heart disease without surgery.

Now that you know all about heart disease and heart surgery, you might be a little scared. Don't be. Heart disease is a serious problem, but it can be cured—without surgery. The Whitaker Wellness Program is safe, it's effective, it's inexpensive, and it can reverse heart disease.

I like to say that the Whitaker Wellness Program rests on the "Four Pillars of Therapy": diet, nutritional supplements, progressive exercise, and, for some patients, a special treatment called EDTA chelation therapy, which is designed to rid the body of harmful poisons.

I also use conventional drug therapy—regular heart medications, such as calcium channel blockers and nitroglycerin—designed primarily to forestall another heart attack while the patient gets well. I would much rather see my patients use this type of conventional medicine than have surgery. But heart drugs are not a cure. A patient who is on such a drug can never be said to be well, and it is wellness, not simply postponing the next heart attack, that we are after. Our goal is not to permanently subjugate the body to the tyranny of invasive medicine but to strengthen the body so it can heal itself.

We begin with a *very* low fat diet to banish excess bad cholesterol and free radicals. In the next few chapters I will explain how and why the diet works and show you how easy it is to stay on such a diet for life. By the way, it does not involve starving yourself. For most patients the goal is not even to lose weight, although most do.

Diet alone, however, will not get you all the vitamins and minerals you need to fight free radicals and the other enemies of a sound heart. So the second part of the program is a vitamin and nutritional supplement regimen: Water-soluble B-complex vitamins, antioxidants such as vitamin C, vitamin E, and beta carotene, as well as number of other special nutrients and "heart helpers."

To this we add a carefully planned, moderate, progressive exercise program. Many heart patients are afraid to exercise and few people always love their workouts. But exercise is essential and there are ways to make it less painful and time consuming.

The fourth part of the plan, EDTA chelation therapy, given intravenously, seeks out and eliminates harmful minerals inside the body, especially heavy metals such as mercury, lead, and cadmium, that harden the arteries and contribute to heart disease.

THEY TRIUMPHED WITHOUT SURGERY

I have used this therapy program to help thousands of patients get better and avoid the heart surgery trap. Here are just a few of their stories.

Richard Morgan

Richard was fifty-five when he had his first heart attack in 1976. He had a double bypass. Within one month, both grafts closed down, precipitating a second heart attack, which was followed by a third two weeks later.

In 1984, he was talked into an additional bypass operation, this time with five grafts. After that he started going downhill. He had chest pain, frequently so severe that he would have to go to the hospital emergency room and stay for a week of tests and observation. These hospital admissions occurred as often as every other month. In 1989 he had another heart attack, this time complicated with significant congestive heart failure. Never in the course of his treatment was any mention made of diet, although he was told to try to lower his cholesterol level.

Richard continued to deteriorate. He was on seven heart medications, including a nitroglycerin patch and extra nitroglycerin to control chest pain. He was unable to walk from his car to his office without chest pain and shortness of breath.

In December 1991, Richard came to the Whitaker Wellness Institute for a one-week residence program. He was taught the value of a low-fat diet, moderate exercise, and nutritional supplementation. Gradual withdrawal from several of his medications was recommended, under the close supervision of his local physician.

I didn't hear much from Richard until November 1994, when he and his wife returned to our clinic. A different man walked through the door. He had lost weight, and he walked with a spring in his step.

What made the difference? He had stayed on the Wellness Program religiously, exercising regularly, eating a healthy high complex carbohydrate diet, and taking antioxidant vitamins and minerals.

Here's an excerpt from a note I received from Richard in January 1995.

"Before I went to the Whitaker Wellness Clinic, I had had three heart attacks and two open heart surgeries with placement of seven 'bypass' grafts. Yet I still had to take a whole handful of heart medications, and couldn't walk 30 feet from my car to the office door without having to stop because of chest pain.

"Six months on the Whitaker Wellness Program and I was off almost all medication, and not only walking from the car to the office door with no pain, but also up three flights of stairs nonstop!

"Before Whitaker Wellness, my co-workers looked upon me as a sick heart patient. Now they have forgotten I even had a problem."

Charles White

Charles is a patient whom I have had the privilege of seeing once a year since 1986. When he first came to our clinic at age fifty-nine, he was being treated for coronary artery disease and high blood pressure. In 1984 he had had an angiogram and bypass surgery, although he had not had a previous heart attack or even any chest pain prior to surgery.

Charles has a very strong family history of heart disease, and his father and a brother both died in their fifties from heart attacks. Given his past history, he was extremely concerned about his own heart health.

I started him on a program of lifestyle change, including diet modification, exercise, and nutritional supplements. He has adhered to this program, and what a difference it has made. Every time he visits he appears healthier. He eats a very low fat diet, takes the recommended supplements, and exercises on a regular basis. He has no chest pain and takes no medications. It is accepted that patients with cardiovascular disease, even those with bypass surgery, generally suffer a steady and measurable decline. Charles, on the other hand, is quite active, asymptomatic, and has excellent cardiovascular conditioning.

He writes:

> I believe the reason I am alive today is because I attended Dr. Whitaker's program. Most all my family deceased before age 65, most in their 50s—father, mother, brother, aunt, uncles, most with heart disease. I knew I had to do something different but did not know what to do.
>
> I first went through Dr. Whitaker's program eight years ago. I changed my lifestyle, eating habits, and exercise. I have kept my weight down, health is good. Dr. Whitaker took me off blood pressure medication eight years ago. I take no prescription medication. I am 67 now, feel great. My wife Judy stays on the program with me. She is also doing great.

John Kenney

John Kenney is an active thirty-four-year-old with no family history of heart disease whatsoever. In early 1994, he began having rather significant chest and back pain associated with profuse sweating, which would come on while he was at rest. It gradually increased over three weeks and culminated in an acute eight-to-ten hour episode of anterior chest pain, difficult breathing, heavy sweating, nausea, and vomiting.

Two days later he saw a doctor who did an EKG and found a massive heart attack. He told John that he was lucky to have survived and recommended immediate hospitalization with angiogram and surgery. John was subsequently seen by another cardiologist who did another EKG, as well as an echocardiogram, Holter monitor, and thallium stress test. He also recommended that John undergo immediate angiogram and/or bypass surgery. In fact, he told him that if he didn't follow this advice, he'd be dead in three weeks.

John dismissed this out-of-hand and adamantly refused to be hospitalized or undergo invasive diagnostic procedures. On the recommendations of his mother, Mary, who is very knowledgeable in alternative therapies, he changed his lifestyle, stopped smoking, and cut out the steaks and burgers. In addition, he started a regimen of vegetable juices and multiple vitamins and minerals.

Mary also went to the library to learn what she could about heart disease and came across my book, *Reversing Heart Disease.* She read the book, called my office, and they flew to California a few days later.

I agreed to follow John on this conservative approach, and he has done remarkably well. He has been extremely compliant about my recommendations, which are essentially the same as his mother's: a low-fat diet, nutritional supplements, and a mile walk a day. I encouraged him to increase his walking to a maximum of three miles a day to improve his physical condition.

When I last saw John in August 1994, he had a repeat electrocardiogram that showed a healthy heart.

I spoke to him in January 1995 and he continues to do well.

Bob Duff

Bob had enjoyed good health most of his adult life. He kept up with his yearly physicals and had routine stress tests. His reports always came back normal.

But then things changed. In December 1989, Bob's stress test showed a significant ST-segment depression. Doctors generally believe that such a significant depression indicates blockages in the coronary arteries and a reduced blood flow to the heart. The next step, of course, is the angiogram.

Bob's deep misgivings about the procedure caused him to refuse the angiogram for about three weeks. But his concerned family finally prevailed and he went back to the medical center in January 1991.

The angiogram showed he had a 90 percent blockage in the midsection of his right coronary artery and a 70 percent blockage in a diagonal branch of the left anterior descending artery, the big one that runs down the center of the heart. The angiogram also revealed that Bob had a "very healthy heart." His ejection fraction was 64 percent.

His cardiologist should have said that with only one troublesome blockage, a healthy heart, and no symptoms, Bob was at minimal risk. Statistics suggest that Bob had a 1:150 to 1:300 chance of having a heart attack.

At best, the cardiologist should have told him to begin a good low-fat diet, exercise, take vitamins and minerals, and get EDTA chelation therapy. At worst, the cardiologist should have told Bob to take heart medications.

Instead the cardiologist wrote in Bob's report, "Coronary artery bypass graft surgery was strongly recommended to the patient. The patient was resistant to proceeding with heart surgery. The risks, benefits, and alternatives of therapy were discussed at length with the patient, and he was discharged home in good condition."

According to Bob, no alternatives were discussed. No diet was recommended, no nutritional supplements were recommended, and the cardiologist certainly never mentioned EDTA chelation therapy. Nor heart medications. Bypass was the only thing the cardiologist bothered to suggest.

Bob said no to bypass and began doing some research. He went to the bookstore and bought everything he could find on heart disease, including my book, *Reversing Heart Disease.* That's when Bob came to me.

Remember, Bob didn't have any symptoms—before the angiogram. After the angiogram, his doctors kept him for two extra days in intensive care for observation, even though he had been told he could check out of the hospital sooner. That's when Bob felt his first chest pain—after the angiogram. He wondered if something strange had happened during the procedure.

When he came to me, I did my routine heart tests. The stress test showed significant ST-segment depression, but Bob didn't have any pain. The echocardiogram showed a healthy heart, and his ejection fraction looked good, too.

Under my supervision, he and his wife began a vegetarian diet. In three months, he lost eighteen pounds. He exercised more, and he began EDTA chelation therapy. Today he's healthier than he's been in ten years.

THE WHITAKER WELLNESS PROGRAM WORKS

Of course there are many more success stories of my patients who have avoided the heart surgery trap and enjoyed vastly improved health by following the Whitaker Wellness Program.

I have included these stories to show that the safest and most effective way to treat heart disease is not to open the patient up and cut apart his insides, but to treat him as a whole person. My Wellness Program includes diet, exercise, supplements, and EDTA chelation. You'll be learning a lot more about these four pillars of therapy in the next few chapters.

For more information on the Whitaker Wellness Program, please write or call

The Whitaker Wellness Institute
4321 Birch Street, Suite 100
Newport Beach, CA 92660
phone: (714) 851-1550

Food For
The Heart

CHAPTER FOURTEEN

The Best Medicine

Just changing what you eat can:
- *eliminate chest pain*
- *lower blood pressure*
- *improve heart function*

I consider diet to be the single most important component of my program for treating heart disease. But many people often find it the most difficult part of their lifestyle to change.

The key to changing your diet is to realize—and emphasize—how many delicious and healthy foods are available. Eat as much of these as you want; they will keep you from missing the items that you should limit or eliminate entirely.

While these dietary changes may at first seem inconvenient, keep thinking how much healthier you will be and how my diet program can help your heart. Isn't giving up eggs and bacon in the morning easier than having bypass surgery?

RETHINKING THE AMERICAN DIET

The American diet, with its emphasis on meat and other animal products, is killing us. An abundance of scientific evidence shows that people from other cultures who adopt our high-fat, high-cholesterol diet soon become prey to the same sicknesses that have plagued Americans for years.

When populations that were largely vegetarian begin eating fatty animal products, chronic diseases that were virtually unknown before begin to occur regularly, including heart disease. The Western diet derives a little less than half of its calories from fat, about the same amount from carbohydrates, and takes in about 12 percent of its calories in protein. By comparison, the Oriental diet takes in only 10 percent of calories in the form of fats, and 80 percent in carbohydrates. The Oriental diet includes roughly the same amount of protein as the Western diet, but this protein is usually in the form of lower fat fish products, instead of red meat and dairy foods. Underdeveloped countries usually have a diet mix similar to the Oriental diet.

As fat intake increases, so does heart disease.

Since only about 10 percent of their calories come from fat, the Japanese have historically had low cholesterol levels and almost no heart disease. But, as mentioned elsewhere, when Japanese move to America and adopt our diet, their cholesterol levels rise significantly, as does their heart disease. Autopsies of Japanese men in Japan and the United States have shown that those who remained in Japan and maintained the traditional diet had no significant arterial damage, while those living in the United States had severe and progressive damage. In fact, Japanese men who lived in America had more arterial damage by the time they were thirty than the average seventy-year-old Japanese man who remained in Japan.

In the light of this evidence, some doctors began paying attention to the link between diet and heart health. And we began rethinking the American diet, prescribing a low-fat diet that limited the intake of animal products. Yet many of the scientific and medical establishment ignored the data and continued to promote a "balanced diet" that included a great deal of meat, eggs, butter, and other foods that are proven unhealthy.

Finally the epidemiological studies began focusing, not on other populations, but on the United States itself. Researchers saw that while we had contained or found the cure for many infectious diseases, there was a great rise in chronic diseases, and they began to concentrate on these diseases and their possible causes.

Researchers began to discover the link between diet and health. And the data proved what many of us already knew: The American diet is unhealthy and the cause of many of our illnesses, including heart disease. Our bodies were not built to consume mass quantities of meat and dairy fats; instead, we should eat vegetables, fruits, nuts, and grains.

WHOLE FOOD AND NOTHING BUT

As far as foods are concerned, the more natural and whole, the better. The best foods are those that haven't been processed, refined, stripped of nutrients, preserved, packaged, colored, or reconstituted. The process of preparing commercial food generally replaces healthy nutrients with dangerous free radicals. Most of the foods on grocery shelves have been violated in one way or another. Americans derive two-thirds of their calories from processed, or "dismembered" foods. But if you're choosy, you can find foods in their whole, natural, and unadulterated states.

Don't eat processed foods when a natural alternative is available. Better yet, make the extra effort to get the freshest whole foods in your diet whenever possible. Whole foods are what nature intended us to eat, and processed foods, however convenient, can kill you.

All foods are whole when grown, and each whole food contains a host of nutrients. But most of these nutrients are lost when the food is processed. Take a sugar beet. The sugar is extracted and purified, leaving us with white sugar that has no positive nutritive value and is bad for your heart. And what about wheat? A whole grain is stripped of its bran and germ (the best parts) to make white flour. When oil is extracted from nuts and seeds, all the vitamin E is lost.

The way to regain these lost nutrients is to eat foods as whole as possible. Instead of french fries, eat a baked potato. Go for whole grain cereal instead of the processed stuff, in which the grains are pulverized and then reformed into something that barely resembles food. Instead of fruit juices, eat the fruits themselves.

Not only does processing rob foods of nutrients, but it also creates dangerous free radicals. As soon as the food is altered, oxidation begins. And unhealthy preservatives are often used to check that oxidization.

So go for natural foods in their whole form, the way nature intended them to be eaten.

LOADING UP ON CARBOS

Your optimum nutritional goal is not only to reduce the amount of total fat, saturated fat, and cholesterol in your diet, but also to increase your intake of carbohydrates from starches. Starches—such as potatoes, pasta, breads, corn, rice, and other complex carbohydrate foods—have gotten an undeserved and totally unwarranted reputation. Complex carbohydrates don't make you fat and don't clog your coronary arteries. Eating a lot of starches might actually lower your weight and clean out those arteries.

Here are some easy ways to increase the starches and other complex carbohydrates in your diet.

- When grocery shopping, head right for the produce section, where you can stock up on potatoes, onions, carrots, garlic, and a host of salad vegetables as well as fruits. Unprocessed food is always less expensive—and more healthy—than the same food after it has been peeled, chopped, deep fried, salted, preserved, and put in a box.

- Go next to the rice, bean, and soup section. There are numerous kinds of beans currently offered. Many of the prepackaged dry soup mixes are excellent; just leave out whatever fat or meat is called for in the directions—which you won't miss at all.

- Add a green salad to your meal. And be sure to eat some raw vegetables every day.

For this style of nutrition you don't need to read labels. Go for the fresh, whole foods, and you can't go wrong.

USE LESS PROTEIN

Your body's requirements for protein are amazingly small. Protein is used primarily for "maintenance" of the body and for the making the millions of enzymes that the body uses every day. But the building blocks of these enzymes and body proteins are conserved and reused, so you don't need to replace them in great amounts. You certainly don't need as much protein as is recommended in the standard "balanced diet."

You should dramatically reduce the amount of protein in your diet, and here are some ways to do that.

➤ Eliminate major sources of animal foods, which are characteristically high in protein. The more vegetarian you become, the less excess protein you eat.

➤ If you are not ready for that, have a low-protein meal at least once a day. Eat a meal of vegetables, fruit, rice, corn, potatoes, or a variety of other side dishes without any meat or other animal products. It may seem strange at first, but if you can get used to it, you will be much healthier, your digestion will be better, and you will enjoy these meals more than you realize.

➤ Or, try eliminating all animal products from your diet at least two days out of the week. On those days, eat only fruits, vegetables, and grain products. Your kidneys will love you for it; so will your bones. In fact, your whole body will rejoice.

QUIT CHEWING THE FAT

By significantly lowering the fat in their diet many of my patients have made truly miraculous recoveries. They eliminated their chest pain entirely, lowered their blood pressure, and improved their heart function by simply making this dietary change.

How do you start cutting out fat? The suggestions I've given you for reducing your protein intake also reduce your fat intake dramatically. You should also start reading labels, primarily to eliminate dietary fat. In doing so, the rule of nine is helpful.

Your goal is to consume foods that contain only 15 percent to 20 percent of their calories from fat. To determine the fat calories from a nutrition label that lists the fat in grams, simply multiply the grams of fat by nine. (There are nine calories in a gram of fat.) This number tells you how many of the total calories are from fat. If you divide the fat calories by the total calories, you will arrive at the percentage of fat. For example, if there are 100 calories total and 5 grams of fat, 5 times 9 equals 45; 45 divided by 100 equals .45, or 45 percent fat.

In the next chapter I'll go into more detail concerning foods and fat.

CHAPTER FIFTEEN

The Right Fats

How to get the good fats you need, in the healthiest possible form, while cutting out the heartbreakers.

Almost all foods, except water, contain varying amounts of fat. Animal meats, poultry, fish, and dairy products like cheese, butter, lard, and eggs are high in fats, especially bad saturated fats and cholesterol. Nuts, seeds, avocados, coconuts, and the oils that come from these substances are also high-fat foods, but these foods have antioxidants built right into them so they're good for you in moderation. Vegetables fats are also less of a problem because they're generally poly- and monounsaturated.

BUTTER OR MARGARINE?

Butter is high in both cholesterol and saturated fats. Does that mean you should put margarine or one of the butter substitutes on your toast? Not necessarily. Although it is generally healthier to substitute a vegetable food (margarine is made from vegetable oil) for an animal food (butter, of course, is made from milk), margarine isn't much better for you than butter. In fact, where the heart is concerned, it's one of the worst foods you can eat.

Margarine damages your heart in several different ways. It raises LDL cholesterol levels, and it lowers HDL cholesterol levels. It also interferes with the metabolism of essential fatty acids. Some studies have even linked margarine with cancer.

The problem with margarine is that the vegetable oil is converted into a solid form by *hydrogenation*. In the process of hydrogenation, a hydrogen molecule is added to the natural unsaturated fatty acid molecule of vegetable oil. Presto: a saturated fat. Hydrogenation forces a hydrogen atom into the double-bond sites and changes the fat molecule from a healthy bent shape, which allows it to be fluid, into a straight and firm shape, which keeps products like margarine hard when they're out of the refrigerator.

To make matters worse, heat and chemicals are used to make margarine, which further alters the molecular structure and thus renders the oil even more harmful to your body.

My advice is simply to do without both butter and margarine. If you sauté your vegetables, cook them in a nonstick pan, with water or broth, not oil. If you must use oil, extra virgin olive oil holds up best to heat and should be used instead of other fats.

The fault doesn't lie only in butter and margarine. There are a lot of similar foods that contain high levels of bad fats, as the accompanying box shows.

FOODS HIGH IN SATURATED FATS

Stick Margarine:	9.9 to 47.8 percent
Tub Margarine:	4.4 to 43.4 percent
Vegetable Oil Shortening:	up to 37.3 percent
French Fries:	up to 37.4 percent
Vegetable Salad Oil:	up to 13.7 percent
Candy:	up to 38.6 percent
Bakery Goods:	up to 33.5 percent

CHOOSING THE RIGHT OIL

Make sure you select oils that are less than a few months old. Look for organic oils that are crude or have been expeller pressed, mechanically pressed—not cold pressed—or nitrogen packed; the label should tell you. Buy oils that are stored in dark, preferably opaque containers and are refrigerated. In most cases, these oils are found at health food stores. Be wary of any others.

Use oils sparingly when you cook, but they're fine on salads and foods that either are cold or have cooled since cooking.

Ultimately, you want a good dose of omega-3 and omega-6 oils because, as mentioned earlier, our bodies cannot manufacture either of them and they're the building blocks for all other fats; also, when your body produces fat from these two fatty acids, it produces good fats.

The following oils are the few that have a fairly good balance of both omega-3 and omega-6, by the percentage listed. Just remember to keep your intake as even as you can.

——— OILS RICH IN OMEGA-3 AND OMEGA-6 ———

Percentage

	Omega-3	Omega-6
Flax	57 %	16 %
Pumpkin	15 %	42 %
Soy	9 %	50 %
Walnut	5 %	51 %

Mayonnaise

Keep away from it.

Most mayonnaise found on grocery store shelves is made from heat-damaged, highly processed oils. The addition of sweeteners, stabilizers, eggs, salt, and vinegar and/or lemon masks the otherwise unpleasant flavor of the oil.

Olive Oil

We have all heard how Mediterranean people have less heart disease, and how much they consume olive oil. Olive oil contains no linolenic acid (omega-3), about 8 percent linoleic acid (omega-6), and 76 percent oleic acid (omega-9).

Because of its structure, olive oil's oleic acid is resistant to oxidation and that's in its favor. But remember, olive oil is commonly unheated when it's used on salads, and Europeans tend to add it to foods after cooking.

Unheated olive oil isn't going to hurt you, but it's not going to help you either. Use it very sparingly.

Flax Oil

Even if you get a healthy level of fatty acids from your diet, it is probably a good idea to supplement with omega-3 fatty acids. Our hunter-gatherer ancestors had a ratio of omega-6 to omega-3 fatty acids of five or six to one. The ratio in an average American's diet is somewhere around twenty-four to one. To achieve a more healthy ratio, you should supplement your diet with fish oil or flax oil supplements. This can help reduce your chance of heart disease, stroke, and other serious illnesses, in addition to relieving arthritis and migraine headaches.

Flax oil offers several benefits over fish oil. It contains more than twice the amount of omega-3 oil, and it's a good source of omega-6 oil. Flax oil is also a good source of lignans, which are special compounds that have powerful anticancer, antibacterial, antifungal, and antiviral effects. Research has shown that flaxseed lignans are changed by the bacteria in the digestive system into compounds that protect against cancer, particularly breast cancer.

Make sure you get enough of these good fats, and stay away from the bad ones.

CHAPTER SIXTEEN

The Healthy Heart Diet Plan

Don't weigh, measure, or count calories. Just head to the healthy aisles in the supermarket and eat all the lifesaving foods you want.

You have probably heard about the four basic food groups since you were a child. Well, as far as I'm concerned, there are just three: foods that are good for you and that you should eat a lot of; foods that aren't too bad for you and that you should eat some of; and foods that are bad for you and that you should avoid entirely.

The following recommendations are not dogma. I know that it is often difficult, especially when traveling or dining out, to follow a diet to the letter. But you should use these guidelines to make decisions about which foods you eat and how often. The most important thing you can do now for your body is to exchange the bad, unhealthy foods you put into it that will damage your heart and arteries for the good, healthy foods that will increase your heart health and make you feel better.

SIMPLE DIET GUIDELINES

My diet is aimed at lowering fat, eliminating free radicals, and increasing intake of antioxidant nutrients. This should be your dietary goal. Forget the bad old days of counting calories, strict menu plans, and portions. Simply change the sorts of foods you bring into the house. You could live very well on these categories of foods alone, and, indeed, many health-conscious people do:

Fresh Fruits

Since heat destroys the fragile enzymes and nutrients that fruit is famous for, it's important to eat it fresh and raw whenever possible.

Fruit is a good source of fiber, of which there are two different kinds. Insoluble fiber is roughage that plows its way through your system, pushing all kinds of undesirable elements through your gastrointestinal tract. Soluble fiber moves through the bloodstream and actually lowers blood cholesterol levels.

The best fruits are loaded with antioxidant nutrients. Emphasize them—apples, apricots, bananas, berries, cherries, figs, kiwi, mangos, melons, oranges, papayas, peaches, pears, and pineapple. Eat a lot of your favorite fruits, but also be sure to keep your diet varied and lively.

Fresh Vegetables

Fresh green vegetables are in a class of their own. Don't relegate them to a side dish—make seasonal vegetables the centerpiece of your meals.

It is hard to overemphasize the importance of greens. Among their many benefits, greens are our best source of magnesium, which we need desperately.

Nutritional scientists have recently been telling us that we actually need twice as much magnesium as calcium. Our bodies store calcium quite efficiently but let magnesium seep out at an alarming rate. Eating a lot of magnesium is the best way to keep the delicate balance between the two in harmony. That means eating greens, especially raw spinach, Swiss chard, endive, dandelion greens, romaine lettuce, butter leaf lettuce, and broccoli.

Another wonderfully beneficial group of vegetables is the cruciferous family, also known as the cabbage family. Its distinctive odor is sulfur, which plays a big role in mopping up free-radical residue in your body. Cruciferous vegetables include cabbage, Chinese cabbage, broccoli, cauliflower, and brussels sprouts.

Two other sulphury vegetables that should be daily fare are garlic and onions. Raw garlic also has a high allicin content. Allicin lowers cholesterol and blood pressure and acts as an antioxidant—but only when it hasn't been cooked. So use it raw, perhaps in a salad dressing.

Don't forget the beta carotene-rich yellow/orange vegetables, such as carrots and squash. And remember to wash fruits and vegetables carefully. Most pesticides are in the skin and can be removed with cold water and a natural bristle brush. Buy organic produce when possible, to avoid pesticides and other chemical agents.

Frozen Fruits and Vegetables

Although fresh is always preferable, frozen produce, if prepared correctly, is perfectly good. The fruits and vegetables are picked, then lightly blanched and quickly frozen. Some of the enzymes and water-soluble vitamins are lost, but many, if not most, will be left intact.

The problems begin after the vegetables have been frozen.

Every time these packages of frozen produce thaw out, even slightly, and freeze again, they lose some nutritional value. Whether your vegetables are a good source of nutrients depends on how long the packages have sat out on a loading dock, how cold the freezer in the transport was, and how cold the freezer in the supermarket was.

A good way to test frozen produce is to shake the boxes or packages in your grocer's freezer. If the contents shake and rattle, they're in good shape. If the vegetables are in clumps or in a solid mass, they've thawed and refrozen at least once and perhaps more often.

Beans

Black beans, garbanzos, pintos, limas... we've been blessed with an abundance of beans. Beans are rich in protein, nutrients, and fiber. They are inexpensive and extremely versatile. Unfortunately, they are also notorious for causing gas. Our bodies lack the enzymes needed to break down the carbohydrates found in beans. So once these carbohydrates hit the intestinal tract, bacteria have a feeding frenzy, and gas is the byproduct.

To cut down on gas, try this. Place beans in a saucepan and cover with water. Add 1/8 teaspoon of baking soda, boil for ten minutes, and soak for eight hours. Then pour off the water, rinse the beans, cover them again with water, and cook them as directed.

If you still have trouble digesting beans, try sprouting them first by soaking the beans overnight, draining off the water and leaving them to sit one to three days. Rinse them several times a day until a tiny little sprout has popped out of each bean. Then proceed with cooking.

Also, most grocery stores carry an enzyme supplement that helps the body digest beans.

Rest assured that as your body becomes acclimated to beans and other high-fiber foods, gas will become less of a problem, though I can't guarantee it will go away entirely.

Canned beans are okay in a pinch, but most have preservatives, color enhancers, sugar, and salt, which undercut the beans' nutritional value. If you use canned beans, rinse them first under running water in a colander.

Lentils are a type of bean known for being easy to digest. They cook in less than an hour and don't need to be soaked. They're meatier than most beans and are excellent in stewlike mixtures, minestrones, and chilis.

Potatoes

White potatoes, russet potatoes, red rose potatoes, sweet potatoes, yams—if you're looking for variety, potatoes have it! Plus, they're very good for you—as long as you don't slather buckets of butter on them.

I recommend you bake potatoes in a conventional oven because microwaves tend to make the skin tough and the inside powdery, and change the flavor. And there's nothing quite so wonderful as a yam that's been baked in an oven until it oozes a caramel-like syrup through a crunchy shell. Eat the whole thing, skin and all. Same thing for sweet potatoes and baked potatoes.

Become a connoisseur of good potatoes. Look for potatoes and yams that are firm, well developed, and relatively smooth. Excessive bumps, ridges, and oddities indicate abnormal growth or storage and will most likely affect the flavor.

Corn

While there is nothing so sweet as a freshly picked ear of corn (especially white corn), you're severely limiting yourself if you only eat it boiled.

Stock up on corn in all its varieties, from puffed corn to corn on the cob. Stock your freezer to prepare for the off-season. The health food store can provide you with natural corn flakes.

Brown Rice vs. Other Grains

Brown rice is perhaps the most easily digested of all grains. People hospitalized for digestive problems are given brown rice precisely because their systems can tolerate it easily.

Wheat, our most popular grain, contains a substantial amount of a protein called gluten, which is what makes bread rise. People who suffer from a serious gluten intolerance, known as celiac or sprue disease, suffer unpleasant consequences when they eat grains. Actually, most people have some type of gluten intolerance that they aren't aware of because their reactions are no more than bothersome. Scientists theorize that the protein intolerance stems simply from eating too much of it—cereal and toast for breakfast, a sandwich for lunch, cakes and cookies for snacks and desserts, pasta for dinner, and the list goes on. Other grains, such as rye, barley, and oats, have less gluten.

Since most grains are hard as rock in their natural state, our bodies have a hard time digesting them. But rice isn't a problem, so eat as much of it as you can, or want.

If you are plagued by persistent intestinal gas, bloating, constipation, diarrhea, fatigue, anemia, general malaise, chronic mucous, or laryngitis, ask your doctor to test for gluten intolerance.

Or try cutting out wheat, barley, rye, and oats altogether for a few weeks. Substitute nonglutenous starches to your heart's content, like corn, brown rice, potatoes, millet, buckwheat, quinoa, and amaranth. If your symptoms decrease or disappear, eliminate gluten from your diet.

A Grain of Truth

The difference between flour and the whole grains from which they are made is like the difference between night and day. Crushing a grain for processing exposes its essential fats to the air and light, which makes the fats rancid. You may not taste it, but it's there. It is possible to prevent, but doing so makes the products almost prohibitively expensive.

Test it. Sample a tablespoon of raw "whole wheat" flour or wheat germ. Unless you paid a pretty penny, the bitter stuff will burn your throat.

For the full benefit of grains, eat them in their whole, unaltered state. Look for oat groats, wheat berries, and whole rye. Some take a long time to cook, but you'll be pleased with the way they make you feel. And your heart will be happy with them.

Luckily, for those who don't have time to cook and bake, there are excellent whole-grain breads for sale in most health stores. These grains have usually been sprouted and baked into a very heavy, crumbly, and chewy bread.

Please Pass the Protein

If you are following a vegetarian diet, beans, whole grains, brown rice, raw nuts, and seeds will give you a sufficient amount of protein.

All whole foods (raw, uncooked, and unprocessed) have healthy amino acid levels without the negatives of meats: excessive saturated fats and antibiotic hormone residue. You don't need to worry about your protein intake as long as you're getting it from the good foods I've mentioned. And you can forget those old wives' tales about combining proteins—the belief that vegetable proteins were incomplete and needed to be eaten in certain combinations. This was discounted years ago. Just enjoy the vegetables and grains in all their variety.

Is Meat Something You Want to Eat?

The best I can do is give you the facts and let you decide.

- A diet high in animal proteins increases the risk of heart disease.

- Animal proteins contain cholesterol.

- Animal proteins are high in saturated fats and are almost completely lacking in essential fatty acids.

- Animal proteins have no fiber, which helps the body eliminate bile and other waste products.

- Animal proteins contain large amounts of uric acid, a waste product.

- Animal proteins produce an acid ash that can cause calcium deficiencies.

- It is far more ecologically sound to produce vegetable foods than animal foods.

THE FOODS WE USE SPARINGLY

If you eat these foods sparingly and properly, they can be part of a healthy diet. But none of these foods is essential.

Canned Fruits and Vegetables

Canned fruits and vegetables have already been processed once, and when you prepare them you are processing them a second time. That means their vitamins and enzymes will twice be destroyed by heat and their minerals lost.

Though not entirely without value, consider these foods second best after their fresh counterparts. And, like canned beans, rinse them to remove added salt and sugar.

Bottled or Canned Juices

Why drink juice when you can eat fruit? Juices, particularly fruit juices, are extremely concentrated sources of fructose, a simple sugar. You wouldn't eat three or four oranges in a sitting, but you don't think twice about downing a glass of orange juice, which contains the fructose of three or four oranges. By drinking juice, you miss valuable fiber you would get in fruit.

As a general rule, drink juices very sparingly.

Raw Avocado

Raw avocado is rich in monounsaturated fatty acids, plus lots of vitamins, minerals, and enzymes. But use it sparingly because you should limit your intake of fats to polyunsaturated fatty acids, the kind found in flax oil, raw nuts, and seeds.

Whole Grain Flours

When whole grains are ground, their essential fatty acids are released from the germ and exposed to heat, light, and air. This makes them become rancid.

Manufacturers of white flour have solved this problem by weeding out the essential fatty acids altogether so they can't go bad. But since the vitamins and minerals are extracted at the same time, the flour isn't much good either.

You would do best to grind your own flours from whole grains. Always store whole grain flours (and this includes cornmeal) in the freezer or refrigerator.

Nonfat or Skim Milk

Contrary to what you hear on television, milk is not the greatest thing to drink. These days it's subjected to lots of environmental pollution. Moreover, milk-producing animals are routinely given hormones to make them produce more milk.

Perhaps more important, many adults cannot digest milk adequately. When milk is not digested, it is broken down by intestinal bacteria, which causes bloating, gas, and general intestinal discomfort.

Even if you do tolerate dairy products, use them in moderation. A little nonfat milk on your cereal, in your coffee, or in cooking is acceptable. More than that is not.

Olive Oil

Use expeller-pressed, organic, virgin olive oil. Don't heat it or cook with it, but sprinkle a little on cooked food or use it in cold dishes for extra flavor. Remember, olive oil is an "okay" fat. It's not bad for you, but it's not particularly good for you either. Olive oil is available in spray cans, which makes it easy to use just a little at a time.

Skinless Poultry

Skinned chicken or turkey is a step in the right direction, provided it's not fried or smothered in a fatty sauce. Avoid duck and goose, as even without skin, they are considerably higher in fat. Remember to cook poultry thoroughly and clean up carefully to neutralize bacteria.

Fish

Since it's low in fat and high in protein, fish is an acceptable "meat" source. The best way to prepare fish is to poach it to preserve its fatty acids. Dry heat oxidizes fats, but moist heat helps protect them. Poaching keeps the heat down with the water, and the air stays away.

Eggs

Egg yolks pack a walloping 215 mg of cholesterol. Since 300 mg of cholesterol a day is about all you want to consume, one yolk would bring you close to your maximum.

In addition to having loads of cholesterol, the egg gets worse when that cholesterol is exposed to air and heat, as in scrambled or fried eggs.

If your day isn't complete without an egg, try eating egg whites.

Alcohol

Alcohol dissolves in cell membranes and makes them excessively fluid. In response, the body manufactures cholesterol in an attempt to bring the membrane back to its proper state of fluidity.

While it's true that studies have shown a link between moderate alcohol use and reduced levels of cardiovascular disease, as well as increased levels of the protective HDL cholesterol, I don't recommend that you start drinking for your health. If you're in relatively good health, go ahead and have a drink now and then. But if you're ill, especially with a degenerative disease, stay away from it.

Nonfat Yogurt

Yogurt is a truly remarkable food. It is milk fermented by bacteria, which give it its therapeutic value. Yogurt raises interferon levels and stimulates the immune system. It helps replenish the beneficial intestinal bacteria that are wiped out by antibiotics. It can even overpower the yeast that causes vaginal infections.

Yogurt has much less lactose than milk. That, plus the fact that the natural fermentation partially breaks down the milk sugars, makes yogurt easy to digest for most people.

Always buy nonfat, unsweetened yogurt with live, active cultures. Some brands don't have them, so look for it on the label. And sorry folks, but frozen yogurt, even though it tastes good, has no nutritional benefit.

Squirreling Away Nuts and Seeds

Raw nuts and seeds are a gold mine of essential fatty acids. Not only do nuts and seeds give you the essential fatty acids you need, they are also rich in the amino acids that play a crucial role in fighting free radicals and building healthy bodies. Eat nuts in moderation, as they are extremely high in fat.

Nut butters are another story. Most are made from roasted nuts and many, especially peanut butter, are partially hydrogenated—stay far away from them.

THE FOODS WE AVOID

Red Meats, Pork, and Fatty Poultry

These foods are dripping with saturated fat and cholesterol, and they are too rich in protein for the human body to handle.

Processed Meats

These are the worst animal products out there, bar none. The meat is second-rate to begin with and then it's ground up and shot full of nitrates to preserve the color. Nitrates can be carcinogenic to the intestinal tract. Processed meats have lots of saturated fat, plenty of artificial coloring and flavoring, salt, and sugars.

Fiberless Sugars

Our bodies are meant to consume carbohydrates in combination with fiber, vitamins, minerals, and enzymes. Fiberless sugars are no good for you. Stay away from them. These include white sugar, brown sugar, honey, and syrup.

Oils

The refining process of all the amber-colored oils you see in the supermarket requires extreme temperatures and chemical solvents to extract the oils.

The heat process leaves the oil full of unhealthy and unsaturated fatty acids, free radicals, deoxidizers, and artificial antioxidants. I cannot emphasize enough how important it is to avoid these oils. Flax oil, extra virgin olive oil, and perhaps unrefined canola oil are really the only acceptable oils.

Mayonnaise

You now know that oil gets rancid when it's exposed to air. Well, what do manufacturers do with oils that have gone rancid? They cover them up with vinegar, seasonings, lemon, honey, sugar, and egg—and voila! Mayonnaise.

Some of the nonfat (not low-fat) varieties are acceptable.

Ground Meats

The process of grinding meat releases iron and copper from the meat cells, and both the iron and copper are catalysts for oxidation. The process also exposes each molecule to the air, increasing the rate of oxidation.

No meat is particularly good for you; but ground meat is worse. We tend to think ground turkey is an improvement, but this is true only if it is not ground with the skin (as it is in most cases). Regular ground turkey has almost as much fat as ground beef.

Frozen Yogurt and Ice Cream

We don't even need to discuss ice cream. You know it's not a healthy food. If you, like so many others, think of frozen yogurt as "the treat you can eat," think again.

Melt that yogurt down and it's not a pretty picture. It's full of refined concentrated sugar.

Fruits have fiber, vitamin C, enzymes, B vitamins, minerals—frozen yogurt has none of these. So eat fruit instead.

Peanut Butter, Nut Butters, Roasted Nuts

Grinding peanuts is the same thing as grinding meat—it exposes almost all the surface area of the nut to air. There are no roasted nut butters that are really great for you, but there is one that's worse than the others, and that's peanut butter. The dampness that surrounds peanuts during the pregrinding phase fosters the growth of a certain kind of fungus that's actually a carcinogen.

Also, most brands of peanut butter are partially hydrogenated—and by now you know to avoid that. The only potentially safe nut butters don't have additional oils, are sealed in dark jars with nitrogen, and are made from organic nuts and seeds—not peanuts. Get them in the local health store if you need a break from whole raw nuts and seeds, which are far better for you.

Egg Substitutes and Margarine

The point of developing these substitutes was to give people the taste they wanted without the unhealthy consequences they didn't want, like cholesterol. Remember, cholesterol became a hot topic in the first place because a great many people were coming down with cardiovascular disease. But these days we know so much more about cholesterol that the substitutes are rather obsolete. We know, for example, that the body produces cholesterol itself in response to free-radical damage, and no food substitute can do a thing about that.

Both egg and butter substitutes use artificially saturated or polyunsaturated fats, which produce free radicals when they're manufactured.

We now know that oxidized cholesterol is the culprit. This advice may sound as if we're right back to square one, but I recommend that if you can't avoid these altogether, go for butter and real egg whites.

Salt

Salt is another one of those foods that's always going to be controversial—because it is so difficult to give up. The controversy swings all the way from those who preach it is an absolute poison, literally "pickling" your insides, to those who say as long as you balance intake of salt with intake of potassium there should be no problem.

Sodium (balanced with potassium) is necessary for maintaining cellular pressure. But you can easily get what you need from eating lots of fresh vegetables. When the balance gets out of whack, sodium is free to leak into cells and cause swelling, or edema.

Lower or eliminate your use of table salt, and make sure you eat plenty of potassium-rich fruits and vegetables. Also, drink more water—2 to 3 quarts per day. By increasing your water intake you give yourself more latitude in your salt intake.

Proven Recipes

Although these diet recommendations may seem a little extreme to some, you might be surprised to see how easy it is to adapt to a healthful diet that can be both filling and enjoyable. In the following chapter I include a sample of recipes from my book, *Recipes from the Whitaker Wellness Institute*, which

I have been using for years, both in my Institute and at home. These recipes are examples of how to eat healthy meals without sacrificing your enjoyment of food.

——————— DIETARY DIRECTIONS ———————

Emphasize	*Use Sparingly*	*Avoid*
Fresh fruits	Frozen or canned fruits Fruit juices	
Fresh and frozen vegetables, especially greens	Avocado	
Whole grains	Whole grain flours	
Beans, potatoes, corn, brown rice	Fresh, raw nuts and seeds, raw nut butters	Peanut butter (which is usually hydrogenated), roasted nuts
Fresh, unheated flax oil (expeller-pressed, opaque bottle)	Olive oil (unheated)	Most bottled oils, mayonnaise, margarine
	Egg whites Nonfat yogurt	Egg substitutes Frozen yogurt (even nonfat!) Most dairy products (milk, cheese, cream, butter, ice cream)
	Skinless poultry Fish	Red meats, pork, and fatty poultry Processed meats
	Alcohol	Fiberless sugars (white or brown sugar, honey, syrup, etc.)
		Excess salt

CHAPTER SEVENTEEN

Recipes From The Whitaker Wellness Institute

Ten heart-healing recipes so delicious and easy they taste good even when I cook them—and how to get more.

A proper diet is essential if you want to get healthy and avoid the heart surgery trap. You might think that in order to eat right you have to sacrifice flavor. Not at all. In fact, you'll quickly learn to love food as it was intended by nature to taste and be eaten. Instead of stuffing yourself with refined carbohydrates and animal fat, you'll be eating a nutritious and balanced diet, high in fiber, vitamins, and minerals. You'll feel better, you'll look better, and you'll live better.

The following sampling of recipes are used every day at the Whitaker Wellness Institute. These healing meals meet the guidelines outlined in this book for safe and nutritious eating. They happen to be my favorites, but there are more than 300 wonderful recipes in our cookbook: *Recipes from the Whitaker Wellness Institute.* For more information, or to order a copy (at $29.95 plus shipping and handling), call toll-free 800-705-5559 and ask for offer #BBD28, or write

Phillips Publishing
7811 Montrose Road
Potomac, MD 20854

My diet is about more than just food. It's a healthy way to live.

Corn Bread

Great with soup, and the perfect thing to dip!

1 c. yellow cornmeal
1 c. whole wheat flour
1 T. baking powder
1/4 c. honey
1/3 c. walnut oil
2 egg whites
1 c. skim milk

Preheat oven to 400°F. Combine dry ingredients in a bowl; mix well. Stir in remaining ingredients until blended. Pour in a PAM-sprayed 8-inch square pan. Bake for 25 minutes, or until done.

Prep. time: 55 minutes. Serves 4

Per Serving:

Fat 19.2 gm	Cholesterol 1.0 mg	Dietary Fiber 5.6 gm
Saturated Fat 1.9 gm	Sodium 75.0 mg	Soluble Fiber 1.3 gm
Mono Fat 4.3 gm	Carbohydrate 70.0 gm	Insoluble Fiber 4.3 gm
Poly Fat 11.9 gm	Protein 10.9 gm	Calories 485.2 kc

Lentil Stew

Try adding fresh tomatoes, zucchini, green peppers, ripe corn, and rice for richness. There really aren't any vegetables you can't add to Lentil Stew. Experiment! With soups and stews, the more you add—the better they taste.

4 c. water
1 c. uncooked lentils
1 medium potato, scrubbed, cut into bite-size pieces
1 large carrot, cut into bite-size pieces
1 T. tomato sauce
1 T. vegetable broth seasoning

Bring the water to a boil and add lentils. Turn down the heat and simmer for 15 min. Add the potato and carrot; cook for 30 min. more. Add the remaining ingredients, and cook a final 10 to 15 min. Serve with bread or muffins and a salad.

Prep. time: 1 hour, 10 minutes. Serves 4

Per Serving:

Fat 0.4 gm	*Cholesterol 0.0 mg*	*Dietary Fiber 2.5 gm*
Saturated Fat 0.1 gm	*Sodium 211.9 mg*	*Soluble Fiber 0.3 gm*
Mono Fat 0.1 gm	*Carbohydrate 29.8 gm*	*Insoluble Fiber 2.1 gm*
Poly Fat 0.2 gm	*Protein 8.6 gm*	*Calories 152.3 kc*

Leftovers Suggestion: Toast a corn tortilla in a toaster and use warmed, leftover lentil stew as a bean filling: place 2 tablespoons in center of tortilla with 1 teaspoon or more of mild chile salsa. Roll and eat.

Spicy Chili

1 lb. kidney and/or pinto beans

1 onion, finely chopped

1 stalk celery, finely chopped

3 cloves minced garlic

1 1/2 t. paprika

1 1/2 T. chili powder

1/2 t. cumin

1 t. oregano

2 c. peeled fresh or canned tomatoes

4 T. tomato paste

1/8 t. Tabasco sauce

2 T. low-sodium soy sauce or vegetable broth seasoning

Cook kidney and/or pinto beans, reserving 3/4 c. of the liquid. Simmer beans with liquid and remaining ingredients in a large pot for about 1 hour. (Keep an eye on the pot for spillovers or scorching. Add more liquid if necessary.) Serve over a scoop of brown rice, if desired.

Prep. time: 1 1/2 hours. Serves 6

Makes 1 1/2 quarts

--- *Per Serving:* ---

Fat 2.2 gm	*Cholesterol 0.0 mg*	*Dietary Fiber 7.1 gm*
Saturated Fat 0.2 gm	*Sodium 45.2 mg*	*Soluble Fiber 0.8 gm*
Mono Fat 0.2 gm	*Carbohydrate 55.5 gm*	*Insoluble Fiber 5.6 gm*
Poly Fat 0.4 gm	*Protein 17.5 gm*	*Calories 298.4 kc*

Laʃagna Florentine

You will slave over this recipe, but it will be worth it. Be sure to use extra virgin olive oil, not only for the authentic flavor, but because it doesn't oxidize as easily as some others. When you heat the oil, keep the heat low and sauté gently.

9 lasagna noodles
1 quart boiling water
1/2 lb. fresh mushrooms, sliced
2 medium onions, finely diced
2 cloves garlic, finely minced
1 lb. fresh spinach, washed and trimmed
2 c. fresh carrots, coarsely chopped
1 T. olive oil
1 c. skim milk ricotta cheese
1 egg white
1 can (8 oz.) unsalted tomato sauce
3 T. grated Parmesan cheese

Preheat oven to 375°F. Cook noodles in boiling water until almost tender. Drain and rinse to keep separate. Sauté mushrooms, onions, and garlic in a nonstick, PAM-sprayed skillet, stirring to keep them from sticking. Add spinach, torn into small bits, and chopped carrots and oil. Cook until spinach is tender, 2–3 minutes, stirring constantly. Combine ricotta cheese and egg white, beating well; add to spinach mixture. Pour a thin layer of tomato sauce over the bottom of a 13 x 9 inch baking dish. Arrange 3 lasagna noodles in dish over sauce. Spread half the spinach mixture in a thin layer over noodles. Sprinkle with 1 T. Parmesan cheese. Top with 3 more lasagna noodles, spread remaining spinach mixture, and sprinkle with 1 T. Parmesan cheese. Arrange final 3 lasagna noodles over top. Pour remaining tomato sauce over all. Sprinkle with remaining T. of Parmesan cheese. Bake for 25 minutes. Let stand 10 to 15 minutes before cutting.

Prep. time: 1 hour, 45 minutes. Serves 6

Per Serving:

Fat 8.2 gm	*Cholesterol 15.1 mg*	*Dietary Fiber 10.1 gm*
Saturated Fat 3.9 gm	*Sodium 210.1 mg*	*Soluble Fiber 1.7 gm*
Mono Fat 3.3 gm	*Carbohydrate 47.8 gm*	*Insoluble Fiber 7.8 gm*
Poly Fat 0.5 gm	*Protein 17.6 gm*	*Calories 301.6 kc*

Rice Raffaele

This recipe came from an Italian gentleman who came to the Institute years ago. We've heard that if you cut the zucchini up small enough, even youngsters will gobble it up.

3 c. cooked brown rice

1/2 small onion, chopped

8 oz. fresh mushrooms, chopped

1 large green pepper, chopped

4 small zucchini, sliced and quartered

2 T. tomato paste

1 c. water

1 T. olive oil

2 T. mild chili salsa

1/2 t. oregano

2 T. vegetable broth seasoning

Use PAM and a nonstick skillet to sauté onion, mushrooms, green pepper, and zucchini. Add tomato paste and water; stir. Add remaining ingredients and simmer for 15 minutes. Stir in rice and heat through for 5 more minutes.

Prep. time: 45 minutes. Serves 4

Per Serving:

Fat 5.1 gm	*Cholesterol 0.0 mg*	*Dietary Fiber 7.5 gm*
Saturated Fat 0.8 gm	*Sodium 89.6 mg*	*Soluble Fiber 1.2 gm*
Mono Fat 3.0 gm	*Carbohydrate 49.4 gm*	*Insoluble Fiber 6.2 gm*
Poly Fat 0.9 gm	*Protein 6.8 gm*	*Calories 260.8 kc*

Sesame Chicken Kabobs

For a fun party treat, try using colorful toothpicks instead of skewers.

1 lb. boned and skinned chicken breasts
3/4 c. orange juice
1 T. sesame seeds
1 T. brown sugar
2 t. grated orange peel
1 t. ground ginger
1/2 t. garlic powder
1/2 t. onion powder
1/8 t. ground red pepper
4 oz. fresh mushrooms, halved
1 green pepper, cut into 1 inch pieces

Pierce chicken with fork tines; cut into 1 inch pieces. In a small bowl, combine orange juice, sesame seeds, brown sugar, orange peel, ginger, garlic and onion powders, and red pepper. Add chicken, toss to coat, then marinate for 30 minutes. Preheat broiler to hot. Arrange chicken pieces on four 10-inch skewers, alternating with mushrooms and green peppers. Broil on a rack in a pan 3 to 4 inches from heat, until chicken is just cooked through, about 8 minutes. Brush frequently with marinade and turn chicken after 4 minutes.

Prep. time: 1 hour, 10 minutes. Serves 4

Per Serving:

Fat 3.2 gm	Cholesterol 45.8 mg	Dietary Fiber 1.4 gm
Saturated Fat 0.7 gm	Sodium 43.3 mg	Soluble Fiber 0.2 gm
Mono Fat 1.1 gm	Carbohydrate 11.9 gm	Insoluble Fiber 0.9 gm
Poly Fat 0.9 gm	Protein 18.9 gm	Calories 154.1 kc

Vegetable Tostada

When you crave Mexican...

2 whole wheat tortillas
2 c. cooked pinto beans
1/2 onion, chopped
1/2 head lettuce, shredded
1 carrot, shredded
1/2 c. green bell pepper, chopped
1/2 c. tomatoes, chopped
2 t. nonfat plain yogurt
1/2 c. salsa

Preheat oven to 350°F. Puree beans and 1/2 onion. Toast tortillas for about 5 minutes. Spread beans on tortillas and add rest of ingredients. Top with yogurt and salsa.

Prep. time: 25 minutes. Serves 2

Per Serving:

Fat 3.3 gm	*Cholesterol 2.0 mg*	*Dietary Fiber 19.3 gm*
Saturated Fat 2.2 gm	*Sodium 606.5 mg*	*Soluble Fiber 2.5 gm*
Mono Fat 3.4 gm	*Carbohydrate 79.9 gm*	*Insoluble Fiber 15.9 gm*
Poly Fat 4.7 gm	*Protein 21.0 gm*	*Calories 422.4 kc*

Western Omelet

1 small tomato, diced
1/2 yellow onion, chopped
1 zucchini, sliced and quartered
4 oz. fresh mushrooms, sliced
1 slice green pepper, chopped
1 t. olive oil
2 T. mild chile salsa
1 t. vegetable broth seasoning
1/8 t. black pepper
4 egg whites
4 pieces whole grain bread, toasted

In a nonstick skillet, sauté the tomato, onion, zucchini, mushrooms, and green pepper. Add oil, salsa, seasoning, and pepper. While the mixture simmers, beat egg whites with a fork and pour onto the mixture, stirring while it cooks to keep it from sticking. (Use a utensil safe for nonstick surfaces.) Cook until the egg sets. Spoon over toast.

Prep. time: 30 minutes. Serves 2

Per Serving:

Fat 5.2 gm	Cholesterol 0.0 mg	Dietary Fiber 8.4 gm
Saturated Fat 0.4 gm	Sodium 595.5 mg	Soluble Fiber 1.6 gm
Mono Fat 1.7 gm	Carbohydrate 37.3 gm	Insoluble Fiber 6.6 gm
Poly Fat 0.4 gm	Protein 14.9 gm	Calories 244.0 kc

Apple Raisin Noodle Pudding

8 oz. wide noodles, cooked and drained

2 apples, peeled, cored, thinly sliced

2 T. lemon juice

1/2 t. ground cinnamon

1 c. 1% low fat cottage cheese

2 T. frozen apple juice concentrate

1/4 c. seedless white raisins

1 egg white

Preheat oven to 350° F. Combine cooked noodles with sliced apples, lemon juice, and cinnamon. Separately, combine cottage cheese, apple juice concentrate, and raisins. Beat egg white until soft peaks form; fold through cottage cheese mixture. Fold cheese through noodle mixture. Spoon into an 8 x 12 inch nonstick baking pan. Bake for 35 minutes, or until top is lightly browned.

Serves 6

Per Serving:

Fat 2.2 gm	*Cholesterol 37.7 mg*	*Dietary Fiber 1.3 gm*
Saturated Fat 0.6 gm	*Sodium 190.7 mg*	*Soluble Fiber 0.3 gm*
Mono Fat 0.6 gm	*Carbohydrate 42.9 gm*	*Insoluble Fiber 1.1 gm*
Poly Fat 0.5 gm	*Protein 11.4 gm*	*Calories 234.2 kc*

Fruit Crisp

Of all the recipes we use at the Institute, this would have to be the most popular.

2 c. fruit (blueberries, apples, peaches, etc.)
1/4 c. apple juice concentrate
1/4 c. whole wheat flour
1/2 c. oatmeal, uncooked
2 T. cinnamon
2 T. walnut oil
2 T. Butter Buds
1/4 c. chopped walnuts
2 T. honey

Preheat oven to 350°F. Place fruit in a PAM-sprayed 8 x 8-inch pan; pour apple juice over fruit. Combine remaining ingredients except honey; spread over top of fruit, and sprinkle with honey. Bake for 30 minutes.

Prep. time: 50 minutes. Serves 4

Per Serving:

Fat 10.9 gm	Cholesterol 0.0 mg	Dietary Fiber 3.6 gm
Saturated Fat 1.0 gm	Sodium 99.8 mg	Soluble Fiber 0.7 gm
Mono Fat 2.5 gm	Carbohydrate 42.8 gm	Insoluble Fiber 2.5 gm
Poly Fat 6.7 gm	Protein 4.6 gm	Calories 269.1 kc

THE SECOND PILLAR:

Nutritional Supplements

CHAPTER EIGHTEEN

Starving Amidst Plenty

*Government RDAs of most vitamins and
minerals are the bare minimum for survival,
not enough to heal your heart.*

Most of the nutrients you need can be obtained if you follow my dietary program and if you consume nearly 100 percent whole natural foods. But it is difficult and often expensive to eat only whole foods, and sometimes it is simply impossible, especially if you travel or have to eat out. Many significant nutrients are missing from today's foods due to agricultural, storage, and processing methods, not to mention cooking. These are the very nutrients we need to counteract the effects of pollution, radiation, disease, and stress. For this reason we have our second pillar: nutritional supplements.

RECOMMENDED DAILY DEFICIENCY

Even if you're getting 100 percent of the Recommended Daily Allowance (RDA) of every essential vitamin and mineral, you're still not getting nearly enough of the nutrients that your body needs. And if you deprive your body of these nutrients, your chances of developing heart disease are greatly increased. If you already have heart disease, you need these nutrients to reverse it and avoid the heart surgery trap.

The Food and Drug Administration created the RDA, a seemingly arbitrary set of numbers that many Americans believe constitutes a healthy diet and supplement program. But they're gravely mistaken. In the case of almost every essential vitamin and mineral, the RDA is scandalously low. The term itself is misleading, since it refers to the minimum, not the optimal daily intake. In fact, the RDA is just one step above illness and death.

FIVE STAGES OF DEFICIENCY

There are five stages of nutrient deficiency. In the first stage, the lack of a certain nutrient causes the body to hoard what is left of the nutrient, refusing to excrete it. If more of the nutrient is not taken in, the second stage begins, in which biochemical activities cease because important enzymes no longer have the nutrients they need to do their job. Then comes stage three: The deficiency is strong enough to produce symptoms. Often these symptoms go undiagnosed or ignored. In stage four, the symptoms are so acute that most doctors can achieve an accurate diagnosis. Unfortunately, this is the stage upon which our RDA is based. The fifth and final stage is death.

So if you follow the RDA, all it will do is keep you from dying of a vitamin deficiency. It will not give you anywhere near the nutrients that your body needs to function properly.

Do you have a nutrient deficiency? Unless you supplement your diet with lots of vitamins and minerals, you probably do.

STOCKPILING NUTRIENTS

Free-radical activity is deactivated by a series of antioxidant reactions, each step requiring an enzyme or nutrient before the next step can be performed. If any one enzyme or nutrient is missing, the deactivation ceases.

Nature has given us a bounty of nutrients in our foods to supply us with these antioxidants and precursors to enzymes. But we can make good use of nutritional supplements to ensure high levels of critical antioxidants in the blood, to offset deficient diets, and to compensate for environmental pollution.

People who supplement their diets with vitamins and minerals have fewer health complaints than those who don't. A high nutrient level in the body doesn't just help the body function properly, it keeps the body from breaking down.

HOW TO TAKE SUPPLEMENTS

Recommendations on which supplements to take will be discussed in the following chapters. Think of them as an adjunct to your meals, and take them with your meals. A handful of pills and a tall glass of water is not the way to go.

Here are some guidelines if you are particular about how you take supplements.

- Take water-soluble supplements with fruits and vegetables.

- Take fat-soluble supplements when your meal contains essential fats.

- Swallow a capsule with each bite, beginning somewhere in the middle of the meal.

- Take herbs or amino acids with water on an empty stomach—taking them with food creates competition and lessens their therapeutic effects.

DON'T JUST SUPPLEMENT

Having outlined the value of supplements, please remember that they cannot take the place of a whole-foods diet. You can't make up for the bad effects of an unhealthy diet by simply taking enough vitamins. Whole, natural foods contain fibers and nutrients that no pill can replace. And it's much better to get your vitamins and minerals from natural sources, because there are probably a whole lot of other nutrients in the foods that we haven't discovered yet.

Mom Was Right: Eat Your Vegetables

We've all been told that eating fruits and vegetables is good for us, but only in the last few years have we discovered just how good. Recent studies have uncovered many health benefits from eating certain fruits and vegetables: the antibiotic-like effects of garlic, the cancer-preventing properties of certain beans, the heart health-enhancing aspects of hot peppers, and the detoxifying elements of citrus fruits.

These beneficial effects are due to *phytochemicals*, which are chemical compounds in plants that protect them from the ravages of the environment—ultraviolet rays, oxygen, insects, and fungi. There are thousands of them, and they are different from the beneficial components of plant food that you know and recognize—fiber, complex carbohydrates, vitamins, and minerals. Although you may not know the actual names of specific phytochemicals, you are familiar with them. They're the sulfur smell of cabbage, the burn of hot peppers, and the irritation of poison ivy.

One group of foods that stands out in our research on phytochemicals is cruciferous vegetables. Broccoli, cabbage, brussels sprouts, cauliflower, kale, bok choy, turnips, mustard greens, and rutabagas—the foods kids love to hate. Each of these vegetables is a virtual powerhouse of protection.

Cruciferous vegetables also contain substances called *phenethyl isothiocyanates* and *brassinin,* which inhibit the carcinogenic effects of chemicals by detoxifying them or rendering them harmless. The phytochemical *sulforaphane,* an isothiocyanate extracted from broccoli, actually blocks the formation of breast tumors in rats. This family of phytochemicals has also demonstrated cancer protection in laboratory-induced cancers of the lung, larynx, esophagus, liver, and skin.

Plant Life May Hold the Key to Future Cures

The field of phytochemicals is vastly underexplored, because the natural components of food cannot be patented. Much of the current research is geared toward isolating these compounds in the laboratory and producing chemical cousins that can be patented and are therefore profitable. Some researchers, however, feel that it's the plants themselves, with the unique mixture that Mother Nature put together, which offer us protection. So, take Mom's advice and eat your vegetables.

CHAPTER NINETEEN

Antioxidants: The Big Three

Nature's three most powerful heart healing "drugs" and how to get all you need.

O f all nutritional supplements, the most important are probably antioxidants, which reverse the biological processes tht cause heart disease. The three most important antioxidants are vitamin C, beta carotene, and vitamin E. Make sure you get enough of all three, because they are essential in your body's fight against free radicals and heart disease.

Vitamin C

Millions of Americans are well ahead of their doctors in understanding how to use vitamin C to avoid the common cold. But vitamin C is also one of the most powerful antioxidants. It prevents the generation of free radicals and is essential to healing damaged areas of artery walls before they fill up with cholesterol. Vitamin C also elevates beneficial HDL cholesterol.

The RDA for vitamin C is a ridiculously low 60 mg. I recommend at least 3,000 mg per day. Studies at UCLA have demonstrated that men taking 400 mg or more of vitamin C have 50 percent fewer heart attacks than men taking 100 mg or less.

Around my house, we keep an inexpensive bottle of 500-mg tablets and I simply take a half-handful (I don't even count how many) several times during the day. Since human beings do not produce vitamin C, we need to ingest a lot of it. Most of the mammals who do produce it manufacture amounts similar to my recommendation, so it makes sense to supplement your diet with the same amount your body would produce, if only it could.

Vitamin C is water soluble; whatever amounts your body does not use up, it will excrete. This means that you don't have to worry about overdosing on vitamin C. But it also means that you have to take your supplement every day, because the body cannot store it.

Vitamin C is catalyzed by copper to combine one-on-one with free radicals, taking them out of commission and putting out the oxidant fire that is raging through your body, destroying cells, weakening defenses, and making you more prone to heart disease. Vitamin C also helps beat heart disease by lowering cholesterol levels. It deactivates the free radicals that cause arterial damage and protects against free-radical-induced myocardial injury. Vitamin C is a natural chelator of metals like lead and mercury, helping the body to flush these toxins naturally. Vitamin C also prevents nitrates from converting to the carcinogenic nitrosamine in the stomach and helps convert cholesterol to bile.

Symptoms of vitamin C deficiency include bleeding gums, depression, easy bruising, impaired wound healing, irritability, joint pains, loose teeth, malaise, and fatigue. Environmental factors, such as exposure to infection, tobacco smoke, pollutants, drugs, alcohol, and stress all increase the body's need for vitamin C.

Vitamin C is also quite vulnerable to oxidation. When getting your dietary vitamin C, make sure the food source is as fresh and whole as possible. Orange juice, for example, should be freshly squeezed. Once reconstituted, orange juice has vitamin C only if some has been added.

The best source for vitamin C is a powdered sodium ascorbate-ascorbic acid combination. One quarter teaspoon will contain a gram of vitamin C, which can be easily consumed in a single glass of juice or water. Divide your vitamin C dosage and take it throughout the day, preferably with meals.

The best food sources are all fresh fruits and vegetables, but especially cantaloupe and other melons, citrus fruits, red and green peppers, leafy greens, strawberries, tomatoes, and cruciferous vegetables like broccoli, cauliflower, and cabbage.

Remember, heating and canning destroys vitamin C, so get your dietary C from fresh foods, and avoid anything processed or preserved.

Vitamin C may cause gas and diarrhea if too large a dose is taken at first. These effects will stop if the dosage is reduced, then built up gradually, and taken two or three times a day.

Beta Carotene

Beta carotene is a fat-soluble antioxidant that is partially converted into vitamin A in the body. However, the beta carotene that is not converted into vitamin A provides the best preventive benefits. Beta carotene has shown protective effects against certain kinds of cancer, including lung, stomach, colon, prostate, and cervical cancer. Beta carotene also protects against cataracts, strengthens the body's immune system, and reduces the risk of heart disease. It combines one-on-one with free radicals to lessen their damage to the body.

Signs of beta carotene deficiency include acne, loss or impairment of sense of smell, dry hair, fatigue, growth impairment, insomnia, hyperkeratosis (thorny skin), infection, night blindness, and weight loss. It has very low toxicity even when taken at high doses for prolonged periods of time.

Although the RDA is a mere 5 to 6 mg, I recommend a dose of 25,000 IUs daily, taken in supplement form. You should also get plenty of it in your diet. The best food sources for beta carotene include carrots, yams, pumpkins, cantaloupes, apricots, and all deep-green vegetables.

Vitamin E

Vitamin E is a powerful antioxidant. For twenty years I have been advising my patients to take at least 400 IUs of vitamin E daily. I recently upped that recommendation to from 800 to 1,200 IUs, based on studies showing that low levels of vitamin E are more predictive of heart disease than high levels of blood cholesterol and elevated blood pressure.

Vitamin E guards against heart disease by preventing LDL cholesterol from being oxidized by free radicals. It is oxidized LDLs that promote the buildup of plaque in the arteries, not cholesterol itself.

A study of more than 87,000 female nurses recently published in the *New England Journal of Medicine* showed that the risk of coronary disease in women who took more than 100 IUs of supplemental vitamin E a day was 40 percent lower than in those who did not take supplements.[1]

In one study done at the University of Texas Southwestern Medical Center in Dallas, two groups of twelve healthy men were given either a placebo or 800 IUs of vitamin E for twelve weeks. At six weeks, the LDLs of the vitamin E users had sustained 55.7 percent less damage from free radicals than the

LDLs of the placebo group. The vitamin E patients remained protected from oxidization throughout the study.

Vitamin E thins the blood, which prevents abnormal clotting. It has also been shown to relieve angina and improve intermittent claudication, which is a pain similar to angina that occurs in the legs while walking. Vitamin E also can dissolve scar tissue and help wounds to heal quickly, it can increase the oxygen in the muscle by 55 percent, and it opens up circulation.

A vitamin E deficiency could result in neuromuscular impairment, shortened life span of red blood cells, a reduction in cell membrane stability, faulty absorption of fats, and an increased susceptibility to damage from drugs and environmental pollutants.

High doses are not recommended in patients with hypertension, or with rheumatic or ischemic heart disease, except under a doctor's supervision.

My suggested dose is 400 IUs for every forty pounds of body weight. The best supplement source is D-alpha tocopherol, without the addition of any vegetable oils or fillers but with delta, beta, and gamma activity. But remember that those requiring the supervision of a physician should gradually work up to the proper dose. Do not take iron within eight hours of taking vitamin E.

It's impossible to get enough vitamin E for its protective effects from food alone. But the best potential food sources are fresh raw nuts and seeds. Wheat germ and wheat germ oil are unreliable sources of vitamin E and are most likely rancid.

Vitamin E can also be used as a topical agent. You can add a capsule to your skin lotion, as it is absorbed directly through the skin and helps protect skin cells.

The Scoop on Vitamin E What you don't know about vitamin E might deprive you of its benefits. Vitamin E supplements vary tremendously and it's best to be informed before buying.

The most common natural vitamin E is D-alpha-tocopherol. But within natural vitamin E there are seven "oily vitamins" (alpha, beta, delta, epsilon, eta, gamma, and zeta). Think of them as E1, E2, E3, and so on. All the Es are necessary for vitamin E to have its full antioxidant power.

Back in 1965, when only three companies manufactured vitamin E, no one except radiation biologists and high-energy physicists were too concerned about antioxidants. Prior to 1969, vitamin E wasn't manufactured with the intent of preserving its antioxidant properties.

Many companies manufactured an artificial vitamin E from acetone and turpentine to cut costs. This vitamin E is still available today and it's labeled "DL-alpha-tocopherol" or "DL-alpha-tocopheryl." Watch out for them. There is no beta, gamma, or delta component in either of them and, therefore, no antioxidant properties.

Most companies add a polyunsaturated vegetable oil of some kind as a filler. These oils oxidize quickly and produce free radicals, which cancel out the vitamin's antioxidant powers fairly well. Synthetic vitamin E isn't an antioxidant to begin with, so the only activity in that capsule is free radicals bumping into each other. By the time you swallow synthetic vitamin E, you're either getting pure free radicals, or possibly a vitamin E with less than 5 percent antioxidant strength.

Whole-nature vitamin E is the most expensive vitamin on the market. But it's the best way to get your vitamin E.

OTHER ANTIOXIDANTS

As important as vitamin C, beta carotene, and vitamin E are, they do not work alone. You shouldn't neglect the other essential nutrients in your fight against free radicals. In the next chapter I will discuss these other supplements and describe my total supplementation program to prevent heart disease.

CHAPTER TWENTY

State of the Art Supplements

Heart helpers to lower your blood pressure,
clear out cholesterol, prevent heart attacks,
reverse disease, and give your heart rhythm.

In addition to the big three vitamin antioxidants, it is important to have a balance of other vitamins, minerals, amino acids, enzymes, and other nutrients. Here are the rest of these essential elements. You need every one of them to have a healthy heart.

B VITAMINS

Niacin (B3)

Niacin helps your heart in many ways. Most important, it dilates your blood vessels, which increases blood flow and lowers blood pressure.

Since niacin is water soluble, there is no risk of toxicity. But

always take it in a well-balanced combination with other B vitamins, unless niacin alone is prescribed by your doctor. Prolonged intake of any single B vitamin without the others could
lead to a deficiency in the other B vitamins.

I recommend a daily dose of 50 to 100 mg of niacin. I use a
form of it, *inositol hexaniacinate*, which does not cause unpleasant side effects, such as flushing.

The best food sources for niacin are molasses, nuts, and
brown rice.

Pyridoxine (B6)

Pyridoxine is necessary for fat digestion and removal of cholesterol from the body. It is needed for the production of anti-
bodies and for the proper absorption of B12. Pyridoxine
allows sixty enzymes to function properly, and is also involved
in producing magnesium and L-carnitine.

If you are on the medication *Levodopa*, ask your physician
before taking a B-6 supplement.

I recommend a dose of 5 mg daily to correct a deficiency, 50
to 100 mg maximum. Even though pyridoxine is water soluble,
excessive doses can cause numbness in the hands and feet.
Prolonged excessive doses can result in irreversible nerve
degeneration.

Remember—all B vitamins should be taken in balanced
doses with each other. The best source is a bio-available B-complex supplement. But it can also be found in brewer's yeast,
which is by far the most available concentrated form of B-complex on the market. If you are sensitive to yeast products, try
rice polishings, nuts, seeds, bananas, avocado, leafy greens,
cantaloupe, or cabbage. These foods are best eaten raw,
because B vitamins, like all water-soluble vitamins, are
destroyed by heat and canning.

ESSENTIAL MINERALS

Chromium

Chromium protects against cardiovascular disease and high blood pressure by increasing HDL cholesterol levels. Many studies have shown a link between low chromium intake and elevated blood cholesterol levels and a buildup of plaque in the arteries.

I suggest a dose of 50 to 200 mcg daily. The best source is brewer's yeast. Other good food sources include whole grains and nuts.

Copper

Copper is a trace element that plays an important part in reversing heart disease. Yet copper deficiency is prevalent for two reasons. One, since copper and zinc interact with each other, high levels of one can lead to low levels of the other. By taking too much zinc without copper, you run the risk of anemia, heart irregularities, and cholesterol abnormalities.

The average American diet contains less copper than even the RDA of 2 mg. Deficiency in copper can result in high cholesterol and damage to the arteries.

I recommend a dose of 2 to 3 mg, taken in a balanced formula also containing 15 to 30 mg of zinc, 200 mcg of selenium, and 50 mcg of molybdenum. The best food sources for copper are nuts, seeds, corn, vegetables, and fruit. But if you are supplementing, be careful—copper must not be taken by patients with Wilson's disease.

Zinc

Zinc is a mineral that protects against iron- and copper-catalyzed free-radical damage. It helps convert essential fatty acids into prostaglandins and promotes healing of the arteries.

Too little zinc can lead to prostate problems in men and yeast infections in women. Too much zinc can be toxic, so at first sign of nausea, lower your dose. Make sure you are getting your copper along with zinc.

I recommend a dose of up to 30 mg daily.

Magnesium

Magnesium is a mineral so important to the body's functioning and so neglected by nutritionists and doctors that I have given it a separate chapter later on in this book. But let me briefly enumerate some of the benefits of magnesium here.

Magnesium regulates how much calcium will enter the cells, maintaining a proper balance. It corrects heart irregularities. It helps to control blood pressure and prevent heart attacks and coronary thrombosis. It also helps reduce cholesterol.

People with kidney failure should not take magnesium supplements. And people with severe heart disease should take it under a doctor's supervision.

I recommend a dose of 1,000 mg daily. Magnesium needs potassium to do its job. Also, it is now known that magnesium is needed in a two-to-one ratio to calcium. While calcium is efficiently stored, magnesium is not.

The best supplement source is magnesium gluconate, the form that will probably be absorbed best without causing diarrhea. Brown rice, millet, buckwheat, legumes, nuts, and leafy green vegetables are all good sources of natural magnesium.

Potassium

Potassium is a mineral that corrects irregular heartbeats. But it must be in balance with magnesium for either to do its job. Potassium must also be in balance with sodium for proper water balance in the body.

A potassium deficiency can cause loss of appetite, constipation, muscle weakness, fatigue, depression, and mental confusion. An excess of potassium is possible only if you take an overdose of inorganic salts, in which case the symptoms would include kidney dysfunction, irregular heartbeat, shortness of breath, seizures, and heart failure.

I recommend a dose of 400 to 500 mg daily. Potassium is more effective when taken with magnesium (a deficiency of magnesium will make the heart muscle unable to hold potassium). Organic forms are the only ones you should take: potassium gluconate, potassium citrate, and potassium aspartate. The best food sources for potassium are fruits, raw vegetables, nuts, and seeds.

Manganese

Manganese is an important mineral. It is part of many enzymes and involved in the utilization of choline, biotin, thiamine, and vitamin C. Manganese is essential to the synthesis of fatty acids and cholesterol.

A deficiency in manganese can result in dizziness and memory problems. But an excess of the mineral can cause insomnia, depression, impotence, nerve degeneration, and Parkinson's-like symptoms.

I recommend a dose of 1 to 9 mg daily in the form of manganese gluconate or manganese sulfate. It can also be found in the following foods: bananas, nuts, seeds, greens, avocado, berries, and beets.

Molybdenum

Molybdenum is essential in producing uric acid and helps eliminate toxins from the body. It also plays an important antioxidant role in the fight against free radicals.

A dose of more than 10 mg daily can lead to an artificially

induced gout. People with high uric acid levels or gout should consult their physician before taking this mineral as a supplement.

I recommend a dose of 150 mcg daily. Sodium molybdate is the most bio-available and least toxic form of molybdenum and usually can be found in a balanced mineral supplement. Food sources include legumes, grains, and meat.

Selenium

Selenium protects against the free radicals that cause heart disease. It also enhances the activity of vitamin E.

Populations living in isolated areas with low levels of selenium in their soil, and thus low levels in their plant food, suffer from a much higher rate of heart disease than those with an adequate amount of selenium. And areas in the United States that have high levels of selenium in the soil—South Dakota, for example—have lower rates of heart disease than states with low selenium. Ohio, for example, is a low-selenium state, and although cattle feed there is enriched with selenium, the authorities don't think it's important enough for humans to require a similar supplement.

I recommend a dose of 50-200 mcg daily, but do not take any more than that. Organic selenium, especially as found in brewer's yeast, is a good source. Toxicity is rare in this form, but do not exceed recommended dosages.

Food sources include brewer's yeast, cruciferous vegetables (cabbage, cauliflower, broccoli, brussels sprouts), celery, cucumbers, onions, radishes, sesame seeds, mushrooms, and garlic.

AMINO ACIDS

Amino acids are meant to work together. And they should be taken together. A primary function of all amino acids is to build neurotransmitters. These are chemicals that transmit messages through your brain and nerves. Research has shown that the quality, quantity, and balance of amino acids is crucial to determine the balance of neurotransmitters in your brain. Taking a single amino acid in excess has caused psychosis, hallucinations, delusions, insomnia, and uncontrollable behavior.

L-Carnitine

L-carnitine is an amino acid that helps metabolize fat. It also improves tolerance to exercise for patients with coronary heart disease and lessens angina pain.

I suggest a dose of 750 to 1,000 mg daily. But make sure only to take the L-carnitine form. Do not take DL- carnitine. Our bodies will produce L-carnitine naturally as long as there is an adequate intake of lysine and methionine, which can be found in most fresh vegetables.

L-Cysteine

L-cysteine protects against copper toxicity and contains sulphur, which is effective against free radicals.

It is a nonessential amino acid that can be manufactured as long as there is an adequate supply of methionine, magnesium, B6, B12, and folic acid. L-cysteine is not recommended as a supplement for diabetics as it can negate insulin effectiveness. It is not to be taken in the case of candidiasis overgrowth as it acts as a culture medium for the Candida yeast. And it could interact with the flavor-enhancing additive MSG, causing side effects. L-cysteine needs to be taken with twice as much vitamin C to prevent the possible formation of kidney stones.

ESSENTIAL FATTY ACIDS

As we discussed in the chapter on fats, some fats are not only good for you, they're essential. Fatty acids are well known as a therapeutic tool for diseases of fatty degeneration, like heart disease, because they protect cell composition. They also normalize blood fats and lower cholesterol. Fatty acids strengthen cell membranes, thereby increasing our resistance to pathogens and carcinogens. They stabilize insulin and blood sugar levels. And they play an important role in regulating blood pressure, arterial function, calcium, and energy metabolism. Fatty acids help your body digest fats, so a healthy dose of the right fatty acids can actually help you keep your weight down.

If these good fats are consumed in excess, they are either burned for energy or stored harmlessly in the body to be used when they are needed.

I recommend a dose of 1 to 2 tablespoons of flax oil, along with a diet rich in raw nuts, seeds, evening primrose oil supplements, and deep-green vegetables. One tablespoon of flax oil also contains 5,500 IUs of beta carotene.

Flax and linseed are synonymous. So, to distinguish between linseed oil produced without concern for its nutritional properties, and oil that is carefully produced to preserve the polyunsaturated fatty acids, many manufacturers call their oil "flax oil."

Essential fatty acid supplementation is extremely important. We have been aware of our need to reduce total fats for years, but now the reality of essential fatty acid deficiencies sheds a whole new light on the subject of dietary fats.

OTHER SUPPLEMENTS

The nutrients described above should be part of your supplementary program. But you might also want to consider these other supplements to fight free radicals and maintain a healthy heart.

Enzymes

Food enzyme supplements optimize digestion and assimilation, and reserve your body's production of enzymes for vital nondigestive functions.

Supplementation of digestive enzymes is especially indicated if you have intestinal gas, acid indigestion, coated tongue, excessive belching, or several food intolerances.

Ginkgo Biloba

Ginkgo biloba is an herb that has been shown in laboratory studies to be up to ten times more potent as free-radical scavengers than the flavonoids found in other plant sources, such as citrus or berries. It reduces clotting and the resultant heart disease, strokes, and other circulatory disorders.

Ginkgo biloba has a particularly beneficial effect on brain function, such as alertness, mood, memory, headaches, vertigo, intellectual capacity, and all aspects of aging.

I suggest three tablets daily of the 40 mg 50:1 standardized extract, or four tablets when cardiovascular and peripheral vascular disease are present.

Coenzyme Q10 (CoQ10)

Vitamins and minerals are not magic, but coenzyme Q10 *(Ubiquinone)* comes as close to a cure-all as we are likely to get. A potent antioxidant, CoQ10 is made by every cell in the body, but production diminishes with age and disease, which aggravates the deterioration of both. When CoQ10 is low, nothing in your body works right.

In a study published in the *American Journal of Cardiology* in

1985, 150 mg of CoQ10 given daily to heart patients for four weeks reduced the incidence of angina attacks by more than half. The researchers concluded that the CoQ10 strengthened the diseased heart, allowing it to reach higher levels of energy before pain or oxygen deprivation occured.

In a long-term study of 126 patients with severe cardiomy-opathy published in *American Journal of Cardiology* in 1990, CoQ10 was found to prolong life by a factor of years. In some patients the disease was eliminated entirely. It can help heart and blood pressure patients get off prescription medication.

Who should take CoQ10? Anyone who has a serious illness or wishes to avoid one. The dose I recommend to my heart patients ranges between 180 and 360 mg per day, depending on the severity of the problem. For the healthy, 30 to 60 mg is sufficient.

Since CoQ10 is fat soluble, its absorption improves if it is taken with oil. In my practice, I use chewable tablets of CoQ10 that contain vitamin E oil and are therefore more bioavailable. You can get CoQ10 from almost any natural food source. Everything that was once living, whether animal or vegetable, and relied on respiration to produce energy, contains it. The best food sources are broccoli, spinach, bell peppers, garlic, most fish, seeds, nuts, and whole grains. Storage destroys CoQ10, so make sure to check the expiration date on any supplements.

OTHER SUPPLEMENT TIPS

Don't Take Iron

Unless you have a clear iron-deficiency anemia, validated by blood analysis, don't take iron supplements. Iron plays a major role in catalyzing free-radical production.1

Avoid Aluminum

While aluminum is never taken as a supplement, we unknowingly consume it every day if we're not careful. Aluminum can be absorbed into the skin through antiperspirants containing aluminum chlorohydrate. Other sources of aluminum are aluminum cans and cookery, antacids, table salt, cosmetics, and some drugs.

Aluminum participates in cross-linking between large connective tissue molecules and enzymes damaged by free radicals, leading to hardening and leathering of your skin. Aluminum has been found in the brain tissue of Alzheimer's victims.

The art of supplementation continually develops as new studies and information become available. What I've given you here is an outline to help you get started.

If you would like to keep up with the state of the art, developments in supplementation are regularly discussed in my monthly newsletter, *Health & Healing*. For more information, call toll-free (800) 777-5005 and ask for offer #END710, or write

Phillips Publishing
7811 Montrose Road
Potomac, MD 20854

CHAPTER TWENTY-ONE

Miracle Mineral

Magnesium: the mineral that heals hearts and saves lives.

If I were limited to one mineral supplement, I would choose magnesium. This little-known second cousin to calcium is far more powerful, important, and therapeutic than almost any other mineral. I do not understand—given all the data showing the benefits of magnesium as a therapy—why most physicians still ignore it.

In my practice I use oral magnesium with virtually every patient, and for many of them I prescribe magnesium injections. I also administer it intravenously for certain conditions, all with good reason.

Magnesium Reduces Blood Pressure

As I mentioned in a previous chapter, magnesium lowers

blood pressure. Some of the more popular new drugs that are prescribed for hypertensive patients are called calcium channel blockers. By altering the access of calcium into the cell, these medications relax the smooth muscle in the artery wall and cause the patient's blood pressure to fall.

Magnesium functions in much the same way—but with none of the side effects. You might say it is nature's calcium channel blocker. Numerous studies have shown that taking magnesium supplements often causes a significant drop in blood pressure.

Increases Heart Attack Survival

The heart attack patient should routinely get magnesium in the IV bottle as soon as he hits the emergency room, just as he receives oxygen by mask. Used appropriately, substantial amounts of magnesium can be given without any toxicity whatsoever and with amazing benefits.

In one study, 103 heart attack victims were randomly assigned magnesium infusion or a placebo. In the magnesium infusion group, only one out of fifty patients died, while of the fifty-three patients receiving placebo, nine died.

Studies show that when a heart attack occurs, massive amounts of magnesium are dumped from the heart muscle. This rapid loss of magnesium weakens the heart and makes it vulnerable to fatal cardiac arrhythmias.

Controls Skipping Heart

Cardiac arrhythmia is the most frightening as well as the most dangerous manifestation of heart disease. Arrhythmia is a change in the time or force of heart rhythm, and for many that is not a problem. But for patients with heart disease, arrhythmias can be very dangerous. Given intravenously, magnesium is a powerful stabilizer of heart rhythm.

In one study at a medical center in Orange County, California, eleven patients with ventricular tachycardia (a particularly dangerous arrhythmia) were given magnesium intravenously. Seven out of the eleven converted almost immediately (i.e., the arrhythmia was corrected), and all eleven patients converted while under observation.

In other studies, magnesium infusions have been shown to eliminate cardiac arrythmias even when the more routine drugs have failed. Infusion of magnesium for control of cardiac rhythm is not only a powerful therapy for heart irregularities, but is also exceptionally safe. No side effects have been recorded in any studies that demonstrated benefit.

HIGH-ENERGY MAGNESIUM

A new form of magnesium supplementation, magnesium ATP, is likely to enhance the benefits of magnesium in heart patients. ATP is the high-energy molecule used throughout the body. A damaged or failing heart suffers a loss of magnesium and ATP, which dramatically reduces the heart's energy supply—and thus its ability to function.

ATP can be "complexed" with magnesium, and given slowly, intravenously. The complex appears capable of crossing into heart cells and replenishing the lost energy stores in such a manner that the heart more or less "jump starts" to a higher level of function. An intravenous infusion in normal humans has caused an increase in cardiac output of 131 percent without increasing blood pressure.

In Japan, magnesium ATP is being used for acute kidney and liver failure. Preliminary reports also show that magnesium ATP is beneficial in the treatment of angina.

Ron, a fifty-eight-year-old lawyer under treatment in my office for heart disease and angina pectoris, was receiving diet and chelation therapy with gradual results. One weekend, however, he had two quite significant attacks of angina. He was given a slow infusion of magnesium ATP, and reported to his physician that for the next four days he was more comfortable and pain-free than he had been in years. This experience has been reported by other physicians who have used this substance in a small number of patients. While it is certainly not conclusive proof of benefit, it is very encouraging.

It is not surprising that magnesium and the high-energy bond ATP are so intimately linked. Magnesium is known to be essential in 325 different enzymatic reactions that require or produce energy. A deficiency of magnesium in any one of these reactions could stimulate a domino effect, thus facilitating or even causing disease. Likewise, magnesium, if given intramuscularly or intravenously, may be a safe pharmacological way to stimulate energy production rapidly, which is particularly important in patients with angina or failing hearts.

MAGNESIUM SUGGESTION

I would suggest the following:

➤ Eat substantial amounts of deep-green leafy vegetables. They are excellent natural sources of magnesium.

➤ Take 1,000 mg of magnesium as a supplement. Excessive amounts of magnesium will cause diarrhea, yet most people can tolerate 1,000 mg.

➤ For patients with diabetes, heart disease, high blood pressure, asthma, or a tendency toward any cardiac irregularity, discuss with your doctor the potential of using magnesium by injection, or administered in a slow, intravenous drip. This use of magnesium is for specific therapy, not for magnesium replacement.

CHAPTER TWENTY-TWO

Back From the Dead

Over-the-counter nutrients that can cure "incurable" heart disease.

C harmian came into my office for a checkup recently. I walked into the room, said hello, chatted a little, gave her a hug, drew a blood sample, and told her to come back in six months. She was in great health.

When I first saw Charmian two years earlier, she was one of the sickest patients I had ever seen in more than twenty years of medicine. She suffered from cardiomyopathy, a severe form of heart disease. For some reason, perhaps a virus or nutritional deficiency, the heart becomes so weak that it cannot pump blood around the body and large amounts of fluid collect in the lungs and throughout the body, especially in the feet and legs. The end result: severe congestive heart failure.

When she was admitted to the hospital with heart failure

and pneumonia, the doctors treated her with standard medication. Then they told her she had only six months to live.

I saw her five months after that. And it seemed as if her doctors were right. Her heart was so weak that she had roughly 60 to 70 pounds of excess fluid throughout her body. I pressed my thumb to her forehead and left a thumbprint in the edema fluid. Her legs were so swollen that the skin was splitting, causing long open sores down the front of her legs that wept clear fluid. Infection in these open wounds would have been fatal. When she wasn't in a wheelchair, she was in bed.

A MIRACULOUS RECOVERY

I told the family that not much could be done, but three things might help: coenzyme Q10, L-carnitine, and L-dopa. I put her on this triple treatment and waited to see what would happen.

Charmian's recovery was miraculous. By mid-December she was up, walking around, and shopping with her family, and on Christmas she helped prepare the family dinner at her daughter's home. She lost 64 pounds of water in eight weeks. Monthly tests of her heart function showed dramatic improvement, as the heart shrank in size and her lungs cleared of fluid. By mid-March she was simply another patient and we would argue about her not exercising enough on her stationary bicycle.

Charmian has remained healthy, vigorous, and active since then. In fact, two-and-a-half years after she was given only six months to live, she underwent emergency surgery for appendicitis. She tolerated the anesthesia and surgery without incident and was discharged in only two-and-a-half days.

Coenzyme Q10: Born and Ignored in America

Coenzyme Q10 is an over-the-counter nutrient. Much of the research on this nutrient was done by Karl Folkers, M.D., at the University of Texas. He demonstrated that it is essential for energy production and strengthens a weak heart, sometimes dramatically.

In one study 150 mg of CoQ10 was given daily to heart patients for four weeks. It reduced the incidence of angina attacks from 5.3 to 2.5 a day. The researchers concluded that the CoQ10 strengthened the diseased heart, allowing it to reach higher levels of energy before pain or oxygen deprivation occurs.[1]

In a long-term study of 126 patients with severe cardiomyopathy, CoQ10 was found to prolong life by a factor of years, not simply by months or weeks. In some patients the disease was eliminated entirely.[2]

This powerful agent is scorned by American heart doctors as worthless. But not by the Japanese. Roughly 10 percent of the population, over 15 million people, are taking coenzyme Q10 on prescription or advice from their physicians.

L-Carnitine: Another Heart Revitalizer

L-carnitine is also an over-the-counter nutrient and acts to transport fat molecules into the mitochondria, the powerhouses of the cells. Like coenzyme Q10, it can improve heart function dramatically in patients with heart disease.

L-carnitine is a proteinlike substance necessary to transport fat across the mitochondrial membrane, where fat is burned for energy. It is absolutely essential for energy requirements. It has been shown in heart patients that, when given L-carnitine before an exercise stress test, the heart functions more efficiently. It pumps more blood, with fewer beats, and with less tendency toward oxygen deprivation. The substance has virtually no side effects and is an over-the-counter item. Unfortunately, most physicians are prejudiced against using treatments that do not require a prescription.

L-Dopa: Also Successful, Also Ignored

L-dopa is commonly used for Parkinson's disease and is a glorified amino acid that stimulates dopamine, the body's general stimulant. In 1984, researchers reported in the *New England Journal of Medicine* that L-dopa was very effective in improving heart function in those with severe heart failure. By increasing the circulation of dopamine in the blood, the heart is stimulated in a beneficial way. I remember several years ago thinking that this was a landmark discovery. Yet I have not found any cardiologists who have added L-dopa to their regimen for the treatment of congestive heart failure. For the life of me, I don't know why.

Start Using Them Today

If you've got any kind of heart condition, start today with 60 to 150 mg of coenzyme Q10 and 1,000 to 2,000 mg per day of L-carnitine. You'll find them both in health food stores everywhere. L-dopa is a prescription drug, so call your doctor.

If you don't have a heart condition, and don't want one to develop, start using about 30 mg per day of coenzyme Q10 if you are over fifty and 500 mg a day of L-carnitine if you are over sixty. If they can work wonders for Charmian, with all her devastating problems, think of the good they can do you.

L-ARGININE, ESSENTIAL TO HEART HEALTH

Heart disease starts when the cells lining your arteries are damaged, making it possible for cholesterol plaque to form. Until recently, it was believed that the damage had to be physical. Now, however, it has been shown that the injury can be physiologic, meaning that the cells are undamaged, but one of their vital functions has been blocked.

Healthy endothelial cells produce a substance called endothelium-derived relaxing factor (EDRF). EDRF or nitric oxide (NO) causes relaxation of your vessels and prevents platelets and white blood cells from attaching to the walls. Nitric oxide is the active ingredient of nitroglycerin, which is used medically to relax the small arteries of the heart to give instant relief from angina or heart pain in patients with heart disease.

To make nitric oxide, your endothelial cells must have enough of the amino acid L-arginine: it is an essential ingredient.

L-Arginine and Heart Disease

In a study of otherwise healthy men as young as thirty, it has been shown that high blood cholesterol levels will cause the endothelial cells to stop producing EDRF. When L-arginine is given intravenously, these cells begin producing EDRF again.

The big news is that L-arginine will not only preserve the endothelial cells' ability to produce EDRF, but will also increase production.

Dr. John P. Cooke, who started researching L-arginine at Harvard Medical School and is continuing that research now at Stanford University, recently demonstrated that rabbits given a diet that included L-arginine had a marked reduction in the start of heart disease. The researchers stated that the EDRF produced by the endothelial cells of the artery itself slows or blocks completely every known aspect of the athero-sclerotic process.

Others have been doing research with L-arginine and getting similar results. In fact, in only four recent articles on the subject by four different research centers, more than one hundred supportive articles were referenced. None of these found any specific toxicity in L-arginine.

L-arginine can cause insulin release and stimulate growth hormone. This could be a potential problem for diabetic patients, but to date there is no evidence of it. And even if these potential problems should arise, they would not be nearly as bad as the known toxicities of drugs that are currently being used for cardiovascular disease.

Being concerned about the potential side effects of L-arginine is like not wearing a seatbelt because it might cause "belt-burn" in a collision.

Because of the demonstrated benefits and absence of serious side effects, I have put my heart patients on 6 grams of L-arginine a day, taken at night. You can do the same, taking it either as a powder supplement or in capsule form.

A HOT TREATMENT FOR HEART DISEASE

In his insightful book, *Left for Dead*, Richard Quinn tells how he was just that.[3] He had a heart attack, followed by bypass surgery that his doctor said would "make him as good as new," but didn't. This led his cardiologist to proclaim, "There is nothing more we can do." This is not unusual; it happens several thousand times a year.

After moping around for months, Richard took the advice of a friend, bought 68 cents worth of cayenne pepper, and filled and swallowed several capsules. The next morning he got up and felt better almost immediately.

That was thirteen years ago, and Richard is still going strong. He studied the medicinal properties of other well-known herbs and launched a company called Heart Foods. As soon as he began helping people with his inexpensive, safe cayenne capsules, the FDA started intimidating the businesses that were selling his products by mail.

When you are "left for dead" you're supposed to stay that way. It's impolite to stumble onto a natural remedy that's several thousand years old, regain robust health, and then go out and tell folks about it. No sir. That's against FDA regulations.

Capsaicin Makes Pain Go Away

Cayenne pepper contains five different capsaicins—the ingredient that makes it hot—and has been used as a generalized stimulant and rejuvenant for centuries. Ironically, those with stomach ulcers are told to avoid it, although it has been used successfully to treat ulcers and other digestive problems.

Capsaicin is particularly helpful for heart disease. Cayenne capsules probably work by acting as a general stimulant and reducing cholesterol buildup. Studies with albino rats have shown that capsaicin increases the conversion of cholesterol to bile acids and lowers the blood cholesterol level by binding cholesterol and bile acids in the intestinal track, thereby increasing their excretion.

I recommend cayenne capsules containing capsaicin to all my patients who have cardiovascular disease. The strength of cayenne pepper is measured in "heat units," which are verified by human tasters. Take a dose of 200,000 to 400,000 heat units a day with food. Taken in capsule form, cayenne does not burn your mouth.

DHEA: MOTHER HORMONE

If you're over fifty years old and want to avoid having a heart attack, you can help lower your risk by ensuring that you have a healthy level of the hormone DHEA.

DHEA is the "mother" hormone produced by the adrenal gland. Your body readily converts it on demand into active hormones such as estrogen, testosterone, progesterone, and cortisone. In addition, DHEA is the only hormone that declines with age in both men and women, and its decline signals a host of age-related diseases.

Increase DHEA, Decrease Heart Disease

Elizabeth Barrett-Connor, M.D., from the Department of Community and Family Medicine at the University of California School of Medicine in San Diego, tracked DHEA levels for twelve years in 242 men aged fifty to seventy-nine. She found that a small increase in the DHEA level was connected with a 36 percent reduction in mortality from any cause and, in particular, a 48 percent reduction in mortality from cardiovascular disease.

Dr. Barrett-Connor and her researchers concluded that one of DHEA's protective functions may be to inhibit the enzyme glucose-6-phosphate dehydrogenase, which triggers the production of fatty acids and cholesterol. When DHEA levels fall, the enzyme system accelerates, increasing production of both fatty acids and cholesterol.

DHEA blood levels are easily measured, and I often prescribe supplementation to bring a patient's blood levels up to the healthier levels of twenty- to thirty-year-olds. I am surprised at how low the blood levels of DHEA are in some patients who are ill with heart disease and other ailments like diabetes and cancer. It also surprises me that so few doctors measure DHEA blood levels and prescribe supplementation. This oversight has more to do with the politics of medicine than with science.

Unpatentable Means Unprofitable

There is no patent on DHEA, so no drug company is interested in promoting it as therapy. Consequently, DHEA languishes on the shelf, and many doctors are under the impression that it is illegal. Though it is not "approved" by the FDA for any specific medical condition, it is without question legal. Any doctor can prescribe it.

But the FDA has cowed most doctors into following its marching orders. And since the FDA approves only recently patented drugs, a highly valuable unpatentable therapy like DHEA is ignored.

I have been using DHEA in my patients for some time now, and with startling results. In fact, I could not imagine practicing medicine without it. There are several products on the market that are promoted as containing DHEA, but they don't contain enough to have a measurable effect on your blood level. Additionally, many who promote the use of plant products often state that true DHEA is not available. This is not so. DHEA is available by prescription from compounding pharmacies and costs about $20 a month for a 50-mg daily dose (which is considerably less than most of the other "cholesterol-lowering" drugs).

Since you are already measuring your blood cholesterol level and your triglyceride level, you should be measuring your DHEA level as well. If your DHEA level is below the average range for your age, I strongly suggest supplementing to bring your level up. I use 50 mg every other day for women and 100 mg every other day for men, while monitoring the DHEA sulfate levels.

DHEA also strengthens your brain function, energy level, and immune system.

CONCLUSION

There are many heart helpers out there, all safe and effective. For some of them you don't even need a prescription. The medical establishment won't tell you about them; they'd rather sell you dangerous drugs and surgery that you don't need. Used correctly, these nutrients and herbs can help get you healthy and avoid the heart surgery trap.

CHAPTER TWENTY-THREE

Healing Waters

Is your high blood pressure due to too much salt—or too little water?

When I was in medical school, we were taught that although your body is mostly water, the water is inactive, just a transport system for the solid portions of the body. Increased cholesterol, high blood pressure, and angina, as well as most other illnesses, such as ulcers, asthma, and arthritis, were malfunctions of solids. They had nothing to do with the amount of water in the body. And for the first twenty-two years of practicing medicine I believed this.

Then I read a book called *Your Body's Many Cries for Water* by F. Batmanghelidj, M.D.[1] He argues persuasively that water is the activator and regulator of body processes and that solids respond to the amount of water in the body. It's almost embarrassing to admit that I could have overlooked something as simple—and obvious—as this.

When you really think about it, high blood pressure is caused by water deficiency. The very mechanisms that are involved in elevating blood pressure are the same the body uses to combat water loss. The sympathetic nervous system constricts the blood vessels, causing the pressure to go up.

What should you do? Since many of the prescription drugs you might take for high blood pressure merely alter your body's water retention, why don't you just drink more water?

Drink More Water

I recommend that my patients with high blood pressure go on a vegetarian diet, exercise, take magnesium and potassium, and reduce the sodium in their diets or balance it with potassium. With these tools I have been very successful in eliminating high blood pressure. Now I've added one additional cheap, easily available prescription—drink lots of water.

Nature's safest, most effective diuretic is water. Sodium, which raises your blood pressure, is what the body uses to conserve water. The body brings hormones into play that do not allow the kidneys to get rid of sodium so it can hold more water in the system. If you flood the system with more water, these hormones will not be activated, and sodium will be washed out and kept dilute.

Standard Prescription

So, my standard prescription is eight to ten glasses of water a day. It's important to monitor this. You cannot rely on your sense of thirst to guarantee you will avoid dehydration. A dry mouth is one of the last signs of dehydration. By the time you feel thirsty, you're already significantly dehydrated. You have to take this seriously and discipline yourself systematically to drink water.

Avoid unfiltered tap water. Filtered water is your best and, in the long run, most economical choice. It's a one-time investment and you won't have to go out and buy bottled water all the time. There are many good water filtration systems on the market. Be aware that some of them remove minerals from the water, and you want to avoid that. You might also want to supplement with extra minerals if you use a water softener or live in an area with naturally soft water.

If hypertension is caused even in part by a water deficiency, artificial diuretics, which force water out of the body, should probably be avoided. But if you are on a diuretic at this time, consult your physician. Don't just stop taking your medications. To shift from a prescription diuretic to Mother Nature's best—water—is going to take some moderation.

CHAPTER TWENTY-FOUR

What About Your Prescription Drugs?

The drugs your doctor prescribed may save your life, but they cannot make you well.

Many doctors will suggest prescription drugs to alleviate some of the pains and symptoms of heart disease. These drugs will not reverse the disease, but they may diminish angina or reduce blood pressure. On the whole, drugs are less invasive and less dangerous than surgery. And in some cases they are absolutely necessary. But they are also frequently overprescribed, with serious side effects and contraindications to look out for. (A *contraindication* means that a particular drug shouldn't be used if a particular problem exists.)

If you have angina, or shooting pains in the chest brought on by any physical exertion, you should be under a doctor's care. If your doctor prescribes medication, you should take it, even if you are trying the reverse heart disease through diet, exercise, supplements, and chelation therapy. But as you follow my

Wellness Program your heart should become more healthy. Under your doctor's supervision you should be able to reduce and eventually give up the medication.

WHAT YOUR DOCTOR DOESN'T TELL YOU ABOUT DRUG THERAPY

Recent studies show that when patients are given prescription medications, only 45 percent of them bother to take them.[1] This rampant noncompliance is usually due to fear of side effects. Unfortunately, physicians have a natural reluctance to discuss the potential, and often nightmarish, complications of their favorite drugs. Knowing or suspecting their doctors have not been frank with them, patients err on what they believe is the safe side.

This bothers me too. Doctors are giving potent drugs without giving equally potent information. According to an FDA study, only 30 percent of all patients polled were warned at the doctor's offices about the risk of their prescription drug.[2]

Drug therapy can be extremely toxic. Adverse reactions cause 695,000 hospitalizations annually.[3] The *Journal of the American Medical Association* reported that 25 percent of all older Americans are prescribed at least one "inappropriate and dangerous drug" each year. All told, prescription drugs kill at least thirty thousand people each year in this country.[4]

Remarkably, the inherent and documented dangers of drug therapy haven't dampened physician enthusiasm or patient acceptance of it as a reliable and reasonable long-term method for treating illness, especially heart disease. Yes, drug therapy is often absolutely necessary. But while your acute problem can be held at bay with drugs, you should not see them as your permanent and only alternative. Instead, take advantage of the reprieve drug therapy provides, and use the time to make yourself *well.*

HEART DRUGS

Three classes of commonly used medication can help in the treatment of angina pectoris. First, I'll discuss those three classes of drugs so that if you're currently taking them, you'll have a better sense of what's happening inside your own body. Then I'll tell you more about what I do to treat heart problems.

Nitroglycerin

Of all the drugs used for any type of cardiovascular disease, I consider nitroglycerin the best at what it does. Nitroglycerin relieves the sudden onset of angina pectoris, and taken regularly can even help prevent chest pains. It can also help prevent heart attacks and lower blood pressure.

For a drug that has been used frequently, and for a long time, in addition to being the subject of many studies and tests, it is surprising that no one really knows how nitroglycerin works. Somehow it dilates the smooth muscle of the smaller arterioles and capillaries. This immediately enhances the blood supply throughout the body, and if chest pains are due to an inadequate blood supply, this helps relieve them.

Nitroglycerin is not a wonder drug. It can relax and dilate the arteries too much. Contraindications include acute or recent heart attack, severe anemia, close angle glaucoma, postural hypotension, and increased intracranial pressure.

With nitroglycerin, the most common adverse reaction is a headache. The headache is caused by dilation of the blood vessels in the head. In addition, nitroglycerin can cause flushing of the skin, dizziness, and weakness. (Different from contraindications, adverse reactions are sometimes unavoidable, and often the drug's benefit outweighs its adversity.)

Recently, a patient of mine was also seeing another physician who put him on relatively large doses of long-acting nitroglycerin for very mild chest pain. This is common. But it can lead to an unfortunate *iatrogenic* (meaning doctor-induced) complication.

The patient took 40 mg of the long-acting nitroglycerin on an empty stomach early in the morning and then walked about a mile and a half to a Rotary breakfast meeting. When he arrived, he was dizzy, disoriented, unable to speak, and weak on his left side. He had had a small stroke. It is likely that the nitroglycerin followed by the walk contributed to his stroke.

Many patients who come to me are reluctant to use nitroglycerin (which isn't surprising since my patients tend to reject drugs completely as a means of treating their illness). Nevertheless, I recommend that heart patients take a small amount of sublingual rapid-acting nitroglycerin before starting any activity when they expect to have chest pain. They should repeat this dose every five minutes, and if they are still having substantial chest pain, they should get to an emergency room, as they could be having an acute heart attack.

Nitroglycerin is given in three forms: a rapidly acting sublingual tablet; a long-lasting tablet that can be taken two or three times a day; or a transdermal preparation, or patch, that allows constant systemic absorption of nitroglycerin through a patch placed on the skin. In the hospital it may be given intravenously.

I urge my heart patients to carry nitroglycerin around in case of chest pains. If pain is a persistent complaint, I recommend the long-lasting oral pill or the transdermal patch.

In my practice I gradually eliminate the drug as the patient begins to improve, but nitroglycerin is the last drug to go.

Nitroglycerin is one of the safest drugs on the market, and it can offer dramatic benefits to heart patients.

Beta-Blockers

Beta-blockers probably reduce blood pressure by reducing the output of blood from the heart. They are called beta-blockers because they block responses from the beta nerve receptors—sensors that transmit messages to the heart to speed up and pump harder—which serve to slow down the heart rate and thereby lower blood pressure.

Beta-blockers also block the effects of some of the hormones that regulate blood pressure. During exercise or emotional stress, adrenaline is released and normally stimulates the beta nerve receptors. By blocking the receptors, beta-blockers reduce the demands of the heart muscle for oxygen during physical activity or excitement, thus reducing the possibility of angina.

Inderal, the first and most commonly used beta-blocker, can compound the failure of an already failing heart. Inderal is contraindicated when the patient is in heart shock or has a very low pulse rate, bronchial asthma, or congestive heart failure. Obviously, if the heart is already failing, administering a drug that further weakens it could be dangerous. In some cases Inderal can even induce heart failure. In addition, beta-blockers such as Inderal may cause fatigue, depression, and impotence.

For the angina patient, beta-blockers can help reduce pain and possibly help avoid a future heart attack. But they should only be used briefly, until the patient has made the proper diet and lifestyle corrections.

Beta-blocking drugs include *Inderal, Corgard, Blocadren, Lopressor, Tenormin, Visken, Sectral,* and *Normodyne* (which is the same thing as *Trandate*). These drugs all have the same warnings and achieve the same goals but act slightly differently in the body.

Calcium Channel Blockers

The newest heart disease drugs causing a stir are called calcium channel blockers. That umbrella term includes drugs like *Procardia, Isoptin, Calan, Cardene,* and *Cardizem.* These drugs inhibit the influx of calcium into the muscle cells of both the heart and the blood vessel walls. Calcium channel blockers help maintain a healthier balance between the magnesium inside the cell and the calcium outside the cell. The medication soothes and regulates spasms of the smooth arterial muscle cells and helps lower blood pressure. The action also seems generally to strengthen the entire heart. So what's the down side? In time there are diminishing returns because the heart's renewed strength gives way to an overall weakness.

Large doses of magnesium seem to have the same impact, except that it doesn't weaken the heart. Magnesium injections were commonly administered to heart disease patients in the 1950s, but they have recently been displaced by patented formulas, even though the more expensive patented drugs are often less effective.

Watch out for excessive hypotension (a drop in blood pressure) and increased angina. There is also a risk of heart attack and congestive heart failure, especially in patients who have recently concluded treatment with beta-blockers.

TRIPLE THREAT

These days it's somewhat trendy to prescribe a "triple therapy"—giving heart patients nitroglycerin, beta-blockers, and calcium channel blockers all at once. Beware: The combination of beta-blockers and calcium channel blockers can be lethal. The idea behind the triple therapy is that the heart will be weakened to the point of total numbness and therefore won't hurt anymore. Sure, the pain will be gone. But then you won't even have the warning pains of angina before a heart attack.

WELLNESS THERAPY VS. DRUGS

You should never unilaterally stop taking a drug.

My advice is that you discuss your treatment with your doctor. Tell him you are concerned and that you want your drug therapy to be a temporary therapy aimed at relieving pain. Talk to your doctor about taking magnesium injections. If you believe he is still overprescribing, get a second opinion, or change doctors. But do not start making up your own drug therapy.

Then change your diet, exercise, begin the vitamin and mineral supplementation program outlined in this book, and start chelation therapy.

In a study by Dr. Dean Ornish, patients taking medication were compared with those who made dietary changes. The diet group virtually eliminated angina, averaging from 10.1 angina attacks per week to fewer than one attack per week. In addition, the heart function in these patients was substantially increased, their blood pressure fell naturally, and they all began to get off their medication. The drug group did not substantially improve.

In a second study of fifty patients that compared a diet group with a drug group, the diet group almost completely eliminated angina in one short year. The drug group suffered even more during the same year.[5]

ONLY THE SICK NEED MEDICINE

One thing is for sure. Patients who are taking heart medications are not well. A patient is totally well only when he can be off all medications, fully functional, and asymptomatic. Well patients are those whose lifestyle and therapies are making the disease go away, not making it worse.

THE THIRD PILLAR:

Progressive Exercise

CHAPTER TWENTY-FIVE

The Easy Way to a Healthy Heart

The right exercise program is like a natural bypass—with all the benefits and none of the risks.

The prescription I'm about to give you, if followed correctly, will help protect you from heart disease; it will also help you lose weight, eliminate insomnia, reduce stress and anxiety, curb your appetite, improve your creativity, tone your muscles, improve your self-image, increase your confidence, slow down the aging process, and just make you feel a whole lot better than you do now. The best thing about this prescription is that it doesn't have to cost a penny. And it can be fun.

The prescription, of course, is exercise.

BUT DOCTOR, I HATE EXERCISE

You don't have to be a candidate for the Olympics to enhance your health through exercise. All you have to do is move more today than you did yesterday.

You can accomplish what you need through activities that are comfortable and enjoyable. The important thing is to keep your body moving, keep your lungs breathing deeply, and keep your pulse rate up.

If you have a history of heart disease, or haven't exercised in a long time, you should develop an exercise program with your doctor. While exercise is an essential element of heart health, you should embark on it gradually, following your doctor's orders. Even a little exercise is better than no exercise at all, but too much, too soon can cause serious health problems.

——————— WHY YOU SHOULD EXERCISE ———————

➤ For every single hour that you exercise, you increase your longevity by two hours.

➤ Activity burns up excess sugars, starches, and saturated fats that otherwise turn into cholesterol.

➤ Activity encourages the formation of the good prostaglandins and helps keep your blood from forming dangerous clots.

➤ Weight-bearing movement helps the body get calcium into the bones, and thus prevents osteoporosis (thinning of the bones).

➤ The heart is a muscle and becomes stronger and stronger with use.

➤ Stretching, bending, stooping, and reaching all use muscles that may be getting neglected in the normal course of life. If you don't use them, you'll lose them.

Exercise also

➤ Produces stronger bones, ligaments, and tendons

➤ Lessens the chance of injury

➤ Improves posture, poise, and physique

➤ Improves immune function

➤ Aids digestion and elimination, even helps get rid of constipation

➤ Increases endurance and energy levels

➤ Helps reduce stress and relieve depression

➤ Improves sleep

And finally, exercise stimulates production of natural mood elevators called *endorphins* and the adrenal hormones *epinephrine* and *noradrenaline*. In other words, it makes you feel good.

EXERCISE AND THE HEART

Today's economy has advanced to the stage where most workers do not engage in hard physical labor. That's good news.

But that means that in the course of a working day we don't get enough physical exercise. And just as a sports car needs to be driven to run properly, the body needs exercise. Exercise helps your whole body; it brings increased oxygen into the blood, conditions your muscles, strengthens your bones, burns calories, and keeps your weight down. But most important, for us at least, exercise helps your heart.

Your heart is a muscle, and muscles get stronger with exercise. In 1953, Professor Jeremy Morris of the British Research Council came out with a study of death rates among bus drivers and conductors in London.[1] He found that conductors had a much lower frequency of heart disease (one-third less) than drivers and only one-half the number of heart attacks.

Why was this? Remember, the buses in London are those grand old double-deckers. And while the drivers sat behind the wheel all day, the conductors were walking around the bus and up and down the stairs collecting fares. It was estimated that the conductors went up and down the stairs twenty-four times an hour. That's the same as climbing up and down the stairs of a two-story home one hundred times a day.

Another study showed that postal workers who delivered mail on foot had half the heart problems of their fellow workers who remained at the post office sorting mail. And railroad switchmen, who are active out there on the tracks, have one-third the heart problems of the ticket clerks who sit in their booths all day. In every large study of workers, those with active jobs had a fraction of the heart problems of those with sedentary jobs.

Dr. Morris came out with another study some twenty years later in which he examined the leisure time activities of 17,000 British civil servants.[2] He found that those who engaged in regular, strenuous leisure activities like exercise or sports had only one-third the heart problems of those who were sedentary. And the more strenuous the exercise, the lower the rates of heart disease.

Since then, many other studies have linked exercise with a reduced heart risk. And if you can spend half an hour a day performing some form of exercise, you can burn 2,000 calories a week, or about a full day's worth of food.

EXERCISE GIVES THE HEART A WORKOUT

Exercise makes the heart work better. A heart that is in good condition gets more oxygen from the blood, oxygen that the muscle needs to stay healthy. Remember that angina and heart attacks occur when the supply of oxygen to the heart is limited or cut off completely. We also need more oxygen as we get older, because as we age, our capacity to use large amounts of oxygen decreases.

When you give your heart a regular workout it becomes stronger and more efficient. A heart in good shape is able to pump more blood with each beat. This means that when the body is at rest (i.e., not exercising) the heart rate drops, because it can pump all the blood the body needs with fewer beats. After you start an exercise program, you may notice that your pulse rate goes down. While the average unconditioned heart works at a rate of seventy-five to eighty-five beats per minute, you should be able to bring that down by approximately twenty beats per minute with regular exercise. That's a decrease in the heart's workload of about 25 percent.

EXERCISE HELPS THE BLOOD

Although exercise will not by itself lower your blood cholesterol level, it does elevate the "good" HDL cholesterol and lowers the "bad" LDL cholesterol. It also helps lower triglycerides.

Regular exercise thins the blood by activating the body's fibrinolysis, a system of enzymes that dissolves blood clots before they are able to cause trouble. So, exercise can decrease the chances of a blood clot forming inside an artery and blocking the flow of blood to the heart, resulting in a heart attack.

EXERCISE MAKES HEALTHY ARTERIES

Exercise increases the size of your arteries, so even if your cholesterol level is high, you can decrease the risk of blockages by exercising. This is not a temporary dilation. The arteries grow in size, and their ability to carry blood increases.

People such as the Masai in Africa, who eat a great deal of

dairy foods but also get a lot of exercise herding their cattle, have shown high levels of cholesterol and plaque, but their arteries are so enlarged by exercise that they often avoid heart disease. And the December 1981 issue of the *New England Journal of Medicine* reports that monkeys who were given a high-fat, high-cholesterol diet but were also made to exercise strenuously showed a great reduction in heart disease, enlargement of the heart arteries, and beneficial enlargement of the heart itself.[3]

A NATURAL BYPASS

Exercise can help give you a "natural bypass" by accelerating the development of collateral arteries. When arteries leading to the heart or other vital organs are blocked, the body begins building collateral arteries to carry fresh blood to these organs. Often there is a race between the development of collateral arteries and the growth of blockages. If collateral arteries can be developed quickly enough, the body can create a natural bypass. If not, a heart attack or organ failure can occur. Collateral arteries have saved millions of people by the same process that surgical bypass offers, without the trauma and health risk. Many studies have shown that exercise helps the growth of collateral arteries. In fact, exercise is the only variable that will accelerate the growth of these lifesavers.

But that doesn't mean that all you have to do is exercise. As beneficial as exercise is, it has to be done in combination with diet and supplementation, and possibly chelation therapy, in order to reverse or prevent heart disease. Each component of my therapy needs the others to work. So don't just exercise, or just change your diet, or just start taking antioxidant supplements. Do them all together.

BEFORE YOU START AN EXERCISE PROGRAM

If you have heart problems or have not been active for some time, you should see your doctor before embarking on a program of exercise. I often recommend a stress test to find potential problems at various pulse rates or exercise loads. The test can point out an oxygen deficit brought on by exertion. It can also show whether exertion will cause an abnormal heart rhythm or drop in blood pressure. The stress test can help you and your doctor decide on an exercise program that will be both challenging and safe. It should be reviewed regularly to update your program.

How hard should you exercise? The key is to increase your pulse enough to give your heart a good workout without stretching it beyond its limits. Try this formula to determine your personal "target rate." Subtract your age from 220 to find your "maximum heart rate." (A stress test will give you a more accurate calculation.) If you are 50 years old, your maximum is 170 beats per minute. Your target rate during exercise should be somewhere between 45 percent (if you are just starting) and 75 percent (after you have gotten into shape) of your "maximum." So, if you are 50 years old your target rate is between 77 and 128 beats per minute.

If you are already on medication for heart disease or high blood pressure, make sure that you consult your doctor about the effect of these drugs on your ability to exercise safely. Some drugs will alter the pulse, and that should be taken into account. Others will lower the pulse rate in response to exercise, thereby negating the benefits of exercise. Just remember that if you are taking medication that affects your heart, be careful about initiating an exercise program, because that's also a therapy for your heart.

Make sure you warm up and cool down. Warming up your

muscles with light activity before exercise is especially important in preventing muscle injuries. And when you're finished
with your workout, don't just plop into a chair. Slow down and
walk for a few minutes, give your body a chance to unwind.
This is the time to engage in more intense stretching, after
exercise when your muscles are warm.

And work out for appropriate intervals. Your heart rate
should be elevated to your personal target rate for at least
twenty minutes. Couple this with a warm-up and cool-down
period, which should include some stretching, and you're
looking at a minimum workout of thirty minutes.

Build up gradually. "Weekend warriors," those who normally
do little activity and then go out for a grueling two-hour game of
basketball once or twice a month, are most prone to injury. Start
with fifteen to twenty minutes and increase your workout time
from there.

Finally, exercise at an appropriate frequency. For optimum
cardiovascular and muscular gains, the consensus is four to six
times a week—not fewer than three, but no more than six.
Take at least one day a week off to give your body a rest.

——————— WHICH EXERCISE IS FOR YOU? ———————

There are countless exercise programs out there, and as
many sports. The trick is to find something that you enjoy
doing and will give your heart a workout.

Any exercise program should have these four factors:

1. It should be vigorous enough to cause an elevation in
   the pulse.

2. It should be long enough per session to be beneficial,
   usually thirty to forty-five minutes.

3. It should be frequent enough to be effective, at least four to six times a week.

4. It should be an activity you enjoy, so you will stick with it.

Pick something that is convenient, don't give yourself the chance to make excuses to quit. But most important, pick something that you enjoy. Exercise is good for you, but it should also be fun. Look forward to your daily workout.

Walking

Walking is perhaps the easiest and most convenient form of exercise. You can do it anywhere and at any time. You don't need any special training or equipment, although a good pair of walking or running shoes is recommended. You can walk alone or in a group. While solo exercising is more convenient, exercising with others can be more fun and is certainly more competitive. It's easy to stick to a program of walking for exercise, even when you're working long hours or traveling. All you need to do is put on your walking shoes and then put one foot in front of the other.

Walking briskly stimulates cardiovascular conditioning and uses many muscle groups. Swing your arms as you walk to get your upper body involved. Walking can be easily incorporated into your daily routine. Instead of driving to the store, take a walk instead. Or park your car a couple of miles from your office and walk the rest of the way. Or incorporate walking into one of your other hobbies, like bird-watching. In bad weather you can walk inside; many shopping malls have walking groups that exercise during slow shopping hours.

Walking is the easiest exercise to monitor in terms of time, distance, and pulse rate. That way you can keep track of your improvement as you walk your way to a healthy heart.

Jogging

Twenty-five years ago there were only a few hundred entrants in the Boston Marathon. Now the event attracts five thousand runners who meet stringent standards to qualify. Everywhere you go there are people jogging in parks, on roadsides, and on high-school tracks.

I'm a jogger myself, and I love the workout. It really gets the heart pumping. And it doesn't require anything more than suitable clothing and a pair of running shoes. Of course jogging jars the bones and stresses the joints, but that can be diminished by running on grass or gravel rather than asphalt. But if you have aches and pains in your joints after jogging, you might want to try walking instead.

Jogging is weatherproof, as long as you're a hardy soul and don't mind getting wet. In cold weather you'd be surprised how quickly the body warms up with the exercise—still, you should wear gloves for your hands and possibly a hat to keep your head warm. If you're traveling, it's easy to bring along your jogging clothes and running shoes and go for a spin around the block. It's also a great way to explore a new place; you can cover a lot more ground than walking.

Stationary Bicycling

Another exercise that is weather resistant is stationary bicycling. It is completely safe, there is not even the minimal jarring impact that occurs in walking, and there's no weight stress at all on the legs. Stationary bicycling is easy to work into the daily routine. You can ride every morning or night while watching the news or your favorite program on TV. And it is very easy to monitor your pulse and increase your workloads gradually. Some bikes have odometers that tell you how far you have gone. Others even have pulse meters that tell you how fast your heart is pumping.

Unfortunately, stationary bicycles are somewhat expensive. And you can't take them with you on a trip. It is also a solitary form of exercise, and those who like the social aspects of a workout may miss the companionship of others.

Road Bicycling

Bicycles are taking over the roads these days, and it's a good thing, too. Not only are bicycles more ecologically sane, but pedaling a bike is a lot better exercise than sitting behind the wheel of an automobile. And bicycling is a lot more fun than driving. It's one of the most enjoyable forms of exercise. You can cover a greater distance than you could on your own two feet, and it is a more efficient means of transportation. If you live ten miles away from your office, you wouldn't think of running there and back every day, but that's a fairly easy distance to cover on a bicycle.

Bicycling can be enjoyed by all age groups, and you and your family can make it something you do together. If you're really serious, you can take long-distance camping trips on your bikes. Or you can just go for a spin around the neighborhood.

The problem with road bicycling is that it is not impervious to weather. If you live in a region with a harsh winter, you may have to put the bicycle in the garage for a few months each year. And sometimes bicycling is not safe, especially if you have to ride on roads that were designed for and are dominated by automobiles. The road-hog mentality is changing gradually, and many towns are creating bicycle lanes or parks with bicycle paths. But often you have to travel on dangerous roads to get there.

Swimming

Swimming is a great exercise. It uses every muscle in the body and its a wonderful workout for your heart. Since there is no weight-bearing stress, it doesn't jar your bones, so swimming is great for people with arthritis or bone problems. It's also a good exercise for those who are overweight, since the added weight doesn't add to stress on the body. In fact, all those extra pounds can actually help keep you afloat.

Swimming is easy and convenient, as long as you have your own pool and live in a warm, dry climate. Otherwise it may be difficult to swim regularly. And it is a very solitary exercise. Even if you are swimming with other people, it is difficult to interact with them while you are in the water.

Aerobic Dancing

Many people are picking up aerobic dancing as a form of exercise, and with good reason, too. It's without a doubt the most enjoyable and exciting form of exercise. Why jog around in circles when you can dance? It's very social too. Men and women participate in large groups together. But you can still keep your own pace and not get left by the pack, as is the case in bicycling or jogging.

Aerobic dancing is very good for your heart. At my Wellness Institute patients routinely record the highest pulse rates with aerobic dancing. Since you have to plan your exercise routine with others, it is often easier to stick to the schedule, especially if your aerobic partners tease you for missing a session. Aerobics is also very convenient; it can be done indoors or outdoors, during all types of weather. And it requires no special skills and very little equipment, just a good pair of shoes and a warm-up outfit. Aerobics strengthen and stretch all the muscles, and also includes cool-down exercises to help fight stiffness and strain.

But be careful about the impact of aerobics. If you have pain in your joints, go to a low-impact program. And pace yourself. Don't get caught up in the excitement of the workout and put a strain on your heart. Remember, the trick is to work up gradually to strenuous activity.

Stretching

When we grow old, we often develop a slow, halting gait and stiff, uneasy movements. That doesn't have to happen, and the best way to combat it is through stretching.

Stretching is so simple and natural that it's often overlooked when one is contemplating a program of physical activity. It doesn't make you thinner or build your muscles, so why even think about stretching? Look at a cat or a dog, or even a child. The first thing they do when they wake up is take a nice, long, slow stretch.

There are only a couple of rules on stretching: Your stretches should be gentle and gradual—they shouldn't hurt—and you should not bounce in a stretch, but rather hold it in one position for about fifteen seconds. That's all there is to it!

Stretching is something you can do on your own; it's as natural as yawning. But if you want to make real strides in your flexibility, seek out a professional, a personal trainer at a gym or yoga class. You'll be amazed at how quickly you'll progress, and what a difference it makes in the way you look and feel.

One last plug for stretching: It's one of the best stress relievers around, and stress plays a definite role in heart disease.

Weight Training

I used to think weight training was for the Arnold Schwarzeneggers of the world. I thought that aerobic exercise was all that mattered. Well, I've learned otherwise. Weight training lowers your body fat, improves your appearance and self-confidence, and wards off age-related muscle atrophy.

In addition, it's something that everyone can do. For the chronically ill or the physically frail, even walking around the block can be an insurmountable task. But most people, even from a chair, can do leg lifts and the like. Researchers at a number of medical centers in the Boston area put this hypothesis to the test.[4] They took one hundred frail nursing home residents and put them on a ten-week program of high-intensity resistance exercise training, consisting of lifting progressively increasing weights with the legs while in a seated or reclining position.

The results were astounding. Muscle strength increased by an average of 113 percent, walking speed increased by 11.8 percent, and stair climbing improved by 28 percent. Several patients who had been using walkers graduated to canes.

Although this study did not specifically target heart function, the fact that it allowed these people to become more active necessarily improved their hearts. It reaffirmed once again that activity, any activity, can make a huge difference in your health.

Other Workouts

In addition to the activities that I have just mentioned in detail, here are some other options: gardening, golfing, tennis, dancing, bowling, treadmilling, stair climbing, heavy housecleaning. *Anything that gets you moving will do.*

Whatever you choose to do, do something. It's vital that you become active. Take at least one activity from those listed above and set yourself a schedule to do twenty minutes minimum, but preferably an hour a day. Make it your goal to enjoy your workout. The important thing is just to get your body moving and your heart pumping.

WHATEVER YOU DO—HAVE FUN DOING IT

Even if you follow all the rules—raise your pulse, work up a good sweat, breathe buckets of oxygen—but hate it, it won't do you much good because you won't do it for long. If you enjoy your activity, you'll keep doing it.

If you are already into some sport, you probably don't need to be won over. This special plea is for those of you who think you hate to move. I'm here to tell you that you can do yourselves a whole world of good with a whole lot less effort than you think. Perhaps you are overweight, have difficulty with your legs, or just don't feel spry. Past admonitions to exercise have left you more depressed than ever. Forget it. Just get up, right now, and walk around the room. That's all there is to it.

THE FOURTH PILLAR:

EDTA Chelation Therapy

CHAPTER TWENTY-SIX

The Cure That Could Replace Surgery

A little known, inexpensive therapy that can cure even severe heart disease in 90 days.

EDTA chelation therapy is one of the most remarkable medical success stories of the past forty years: It's also one of the least known. Chelation has been ignored (and worse) by the medical establishment, which is why the treatment is not as popular as it should be. If chelation therapy were widely prescribed, the amount of heart disease in this country would drop dramatically. Invasive heart surgery could be eliminated in all but the most severe cases. Perhaps that's why the medical community is paying so little attention to this wonderful treatment.

Chelation is painless, noninvasive, and administered in a doctor's office. It has been proven to reverse heart disease, reduce blood pressure, prevent heart attacks and strokes, and relieve angina. In addition, chelation patients have reported that the therapy has improved sexual function, increased vision, and reduced symptoms of a whole host of diseases, including arthritis, multiple sclerosis, Parkinson's disease, and psoriasis. There's also evidence that EDTA chelation can help prevent Alzheimer's disease by removing aluminum from the brain, which is thought by some researchers to be the cause of that illness.

EDTA CHELATION THERAPY—THE HISTORY

EDTA (ethylene diamine tetracidic acid) is a proteinlike molecule (a synthetic protein) that binds to metal ions such as lead, mercury, and calcium and makes them soluble in the blood. That allows the kidneys to eliminate them from the body. It has always been a primary therapy for heavy metal poisoning.

EDTA is slowly introduced into the bloodstream where it latches onto heavy toxic metals in the body, which are eventually excreted along with the EDTA. Organic scientists have used the chemical process of chelation for years in manufacturing many different products, from paint to petroleum.

At the end of World War II, EDTA chelation was introduced as a medical therapy to treat arsenic and lead poisoning. Sailors who were poisoned after absorbing the lead paint used on ships were treated with chelation. Not only were they cured of lead poisoning, they miraculously recovered from cardiovascular diseases as well.

Because the improvements experienced by these men were observed but not necessarily intended, chelation was a discovered therapy, not a devised one. It was never proposed as a therapy for cardiovascular disorders; nevertheless, men with such disorders spontaneously improved when they received the therapy for removal of heavy metals.

Back in the early 1950s, Dr. Norman Clarke thought that

since calcium was deposited in the cholesterol plaque plugging the arteries, it stood to reason that EDTA (which also binds with, and removes, calcium) could soften and perhaps lead to a reversal of the cholesterol deposits. He tried it, and it worked like a charm.

Dr. Clarke published several reports on 286 patients with either chest pain or leg pain from blocked arteries, showing that twenty intravenous infusions of EDTA alleviated the symptoms and significantly improved the blood flow in over 80 percent of the patients. His summary in the *American Journal of Cardiology* (August 1960) stated:

"An accumulated experience with several hundred patients has demonstrated that the overall relief from the manifestations of occlusive vascular disease has been superior to that obtained with other methods...

"There has been significant relief in 87 percent of a large series of patients with angina pectoris, few recurrences of symptoms, and a significant lowering of previously reported mortality rates."[1]

Chelation fell in disfavor in the mid-1960s—not because it was proven ineffective, but because the drug patent had run out, leaving Abbott Laboratories with no incentive to "prove" what had been observed. Second, surgery for heart and vessel diseases was on the rise, and EDTA chelation therapy—a relatively inexpensive, outpatient office procedure—was certainly less interesting.

But a small group of physicians recognized the benefits of EDTA chelation therapy and continued to use it and study its benefits. The good news spread by word of mouth from those who felt that they had benefited. It has now been used worldwide in close to one million patients with cardiovascular disease.

A recently published study retrospectively analyzed the effects of EDTA chelation therapy on 2,870 patients suffering from a variety of degenerative diseases. The authors reported: "Using qualitative, but nevertheless standardized criteria for improvement, our analysis showed that EDTA chelation therapy resulted in marked improvement in 76.89% and good improvement in 16.56% of patients with ischemic heart disease."[2]

In addition, marked improvement was recorded in 91 percent and good improvement in 76 percent of patients with peripheral vascular disease and intermittent claudication (angina of the legs). The authors pointed out that these beneficial results could not be due solely to the placebo effect.

Then a double-blind, placebo-controlled trial was done in which chelation therapy was compared with a placebo for intermittent claudication. Ten patients with significant leg pain were randomly assigned to receive either EDTA chelation therapy or a placebo. A total of twenty infusions was planned for the study. But after only ten infusions the patients receiving the EDTA had improved so much that those receiving the placebo were given ten infusions of EDTA as well. Both groups improved dramatically.[3]

HOW DOES IT WORK?

EDTA is a synthetic protein that is drawn to metal ions such as copper, iron, mercury, and lead. The EDTA is administered via intravenous infusion, and, once in the bloodstream, its molecules attach to metal ions, drawing them out of the tissues in the body. The EDTA molecule is then, very simply, excreted along with the heavy metal.

These toxic heavy metal ions play an extremely active role in the process of free-radical pathology. They act as potent catalysts in lipid oxidation, which we are now discovering is the culprit in not only cardiovascular but many degenerative diseases. They also increase the production of free radicals. Removing the metal ions interrupts the process of free-radical damage and fosters normal healing. By eliminating the root cause of arterial damage, EDTA chelation therapy serves as the basis for the ensuing natural healing.

In reducing free-radical activity, EDTA restores prostaglandin hormone balance, which is responsible for preventing arterial spasms, blood clotting, plaque formation, and inflammation. While EDTA protects cell membranes from further free-radical damage, it also helps restore the natural calcium-magnesium balance that facilitates the normal contraction and relaxation of all muscles.

EDTA also restores the body's normal enzyme functions by removing heavy metals like lead and mercury that interfere with those functions. And it binds to copper and iron, which are partially responsible for converting cholesterol into a damaging substance.

EDTA, SAFE AND EFFECTIVE

In 1989 the FDA began scientifically controlled trials of EDTA chelation therapy, and while the results have yet to be released, the FDA concluded that "safety was not an issue" with EDTA. Over the past thirty years, approximately 600,000 patients have had about 12 million EDTA infusions in this country, and the FDA could find no evidence of any significant toxicity. In fact, no fatalities from EDTA chelation have occurred when the treatment was properly administered and supervised.

ALTERNATIVE TO SURGERY

Richard, a fifty-eight-year-old man from England, began having severe chest pains while walking his dog. He was hospitalized, underwent an angiogram, and was told that his arteries were so severely blocked that it would be too dangerous for him to leave the hospital. Only immediate bypass surgery would save him.

He asked his cardiologist about the alternatives to surgery and the cardiologist said, "There are no alternatives." This was all Richard needed to hear to check out of the hospital and seek alternative treatment.

His initial stress test brought on pain within two minutes and had to be stopped at four minutes. After twenty infusions of EDTA, his pain was completely eliminated and, on a repeat stress test, Richard was able to walk for almost ten minutes at a far higher workload with no pain at all.

Thomas, a sixty-four-year-old man, had multiple problems. He had calcium in his aortic valve, numerous blockages in his heart arteries, and a 70 percent blockage in the left carotid artery going to his brain. He was told that he was a "walking time bomb" (this phrase was in his medical records) and that unless he had his aortic valve replaced and bypass surgery, he would surely die. Other doctors also felt that the blockage in his neck would progress and he would need surgery there as well.

Tom decided to give EDTA chelation therapy a try before getting cut from stem to stern.

After twenty treatments, carotid ultrasound showed that the 70 percent blockage in his neck had reversed down to 15 percent, the calcification in his aortic valve had dissolved, valve function had improved, and he was able to walk almost twice as far on the exercise treadmill.

Both men avoided the knife and have improved so much that they are no longer candidates for surgery.

TWO PROBLEMS

The two biggest problems concerning chelation have nothing to do with the safety or efficacy of the treatment itself but stem from the medical establishment's refusal to accept it as a valid therapy. The first problem is finding a doctor to do it; this is easing because more and more doctors are becoming aware of EDTA chelation and beginning to administer it. The second problem is having to pay for it because insurance and Medicare won't reimburse you.

On the first count, I advise you to contact the American College of Advancement in Medicine (ACAM):

ACAM
P.O. Box 3427
Laguna Hills, CA 92653

The ACAM provides training for physicians in chelation therapy and certifies those who qualify. The organization also holds biannual conferences, which provide the latest findings and procedures in chelation therapy and other forms of preventive nutritional medicine. It can refer you to a doctor in your area.

The second obstacle is easier to accept if you realize that bypass surgery costs $30,000 (and it can kill you). Chelation costs about $3,000. And it will make you healthier. By using EDTA, diet, and supplementation, you can probably reverse your cardiovascular disease and its symptoms; by contrast, with surgical methods you can look forward to further debilitation.

The Fetzer Foundation of Kalamazoo, Michigan, which supports research into EDTA therapy, cites another example of this ridiculous policy. "A woman, who had gangrene in one leg, was advised by several physicians that amputation was the only available option. Yet, after her leg was saved by chelation therapy, the medical carrier would not cover the $4,000 cost of chelation, but would have been willing to pay $15,000 if she had had her leg amputated."[4]

One can only hope that someday the medical establishment will acknowledge the value of EDTA and other alternative therapies and, as a result, insurance companies and the government will reimburse patients who choose it.

THE EASY PART

Once you've found a doctor who will administer chelation treatments, the easy part begins. You relax in a comfortable chair and either chat with other patients or watch a movie.

Chelation uses a 25-gauge needle. It's tiny and relatively painless. It's small so that the EDTA solution can drip for three or four hours, preventing excess burden to the kidneys, which later excrete the EDTA with the metal ions.

The one and only big danger of EDTA is administering it too often or too fast. Reports of kidney damage or death are known to have been caused by excessive doses, or by the patient's existing kidney disease or heavy metal toxicity. But don't be alarmed; there have been no fatalities from EDTA chelation when the treatment was properly administered and supervised. The doctors who use it know all about EDTA, so careful administration is standard, making it one of the safest therapies available.

The contents of the chelation bottle dripping into your arm is a mixture of natural vitamins; minerals, including magnesium; Procain, an anesthetic; sodium bicarbonate; and EDTA molecules. Due to the chemistry of EDTA, when it combines with the magnesium in the bottle it releases hydrogen ions that can cause a burning sensation at the site of the needle's insertion. The Procaine is added to dull the burn. The sodium bicarbonate does the same thing in a different way.

Calculating Your Exact Dose of EDTA

Some doctors do a finger-stick test before each treatment; others do a blood draw every fourth or fifth time. Using a little math and the reading they get on your kidneys and liver, plus your body weight, your doctor will calculate the proper EDTA dose for you. The blood tests are imperative because for EDTA to be a completely safe therapy, your kidneys and liver must be able to excrete the EDTA after it has picked up the metal ions.

Number of Treatments

How many treatments will you need? The range could be anywhere from ten to a hundred, and the norm is around twenty-five. Different people need different levels of treatment.

EDTA DOES NOT STAND ALONE

Your doctor will probably urge you to follow other therapies that enhance the progress of chelation, for example, a shot of vitamin B12, and maybe a shot of adenosine triphosphate (ATP), which gives your cells energy. These two shots would act as a pick-me-up because chelation can be a bit draining.

You should also eat healthy foods for the maximum benefits of EDTA chelation. The therapy works best in conjunction with a diet high in nutrients and low in fat. The diet that I have suggested previously is perfectly good if you are undergoing chelation therapy.

MAINTENANCE

When you and your doctor are satisfied with the level of improvement you have achieved (most people feel their greatest improvement approximately ninety days following their last treatment), you will want to set up a maintenance schedule. Typically this means treatment once a month. It's a breeze and you'll feel great.

CHAPTER TWENTY-SEVEN

The
Healing Mind

Depression is part of every disease, including heart disease. To fight it, enlist your spirit in the healing process.

Now you've embarked on a program for heart health. You're eating right. You're getting regular exercise. You're taking antioxidant supplements. You're even scheduled for EDTA chelation. But there's one more kind of therapy I hope you'll consider.

When I evaluate a patient, I pay close attention to his mood and treat it as vigorously as I would any "physical" illness. As depression becomes an even more common and serious problem in this country, mood becomes even more important to medicine. Depression is a disease in itself, but it's part of every other disease as well, including heart disease.

I personally believe that a state of "almost always happy" should be the norm. Optimism and enthusiasm are essential to the survival of the species. If depression and lethargy were the dominant mood, the species would never have survived back when times were really difficult hundreds of thousands of years ago.

So, what can you do to feel better?

First, understand that persistent clinical depression is primarily biochemical, not psychological. Your mood is determined by the concentration of various neurotransmitters in the brain. These substances either lift or depress the mood. The two dominant ones are dopamine (the psychic energizer) and serotonin (the psychic relaxer). The system, of course, is more complex (particularly the actions of serotonin), but in general this description holds true.

Manipulating these neurotransmitters to generate a more positive combination is now, and always will be, the best formula for elevating mood.

My basic suggestions for elevating mood are the same as those for heart disease. Get regular physical exercise. Practice good nutrition. Take vitamin and mineral supplements. In addition, you may want to have your thyroid function assessed, especially if you have a history of cold hands and feet, weight gain, and generalized fatigue.

You Won't Regret a Pet

Another great way to reduce stress and lift your spirits is to get a pet. If you have no preference, I would suggest a dog— 10 to 20 pounds is a good size.

Pets have been a part of human culture throughout history, and in American households, pets are more common than children.

Pets promote health—and this is not a new idea. In 1792 animals were used in treating mental patients at York Retreat in England. In 1919, the U.S. secretary of the interior suggested to the superintendent of St. Elizabeth's Hospital in Washington, D.C., that dogs be used as companions for psychiatric patients.

Researchers are now documenting that "pet therapy" works; in fact, pets can save lives.

In ninety-two consecutive heart attack patients discharged from a coronary care unit, thirty-nine were petless and fifty-three had pets. The one-year mortality rate in the petless group was 28 percent, compared with only 6 percent among those who had pets.[1] Interaction with pets has been shown to lower blood pressure and heart rate, subtle changes that can have enormous health benefits.

A recent study at UCLA found that Medicare patients who have pets visit their doctor much less frequently and seem to tolerate stressful events better.[2] In another study, new pet owners reported substantial improvements in their health, sense of security, and amount of exercise. New dog owners fared better than cat owners because they got more exercise. People who would not take a walk for their own health or enjoyment routinely did for their dogs.

CARING IS HEALING

Ironically, the most common reason people give for not having pets—having to care for them—is one of the reasons pets improve health. Pets make you "extend" yourself when you normally wouldn't. Pets turn people who are ill, or just want better health, from "care receivers" to "care givers." If you put a small pet on the lap of a severely arthritic patient, the otherwise motionless patient will move to stroke the animal.

Caring for a pet is only part of the story; after all, you care for your car. It is the relationship that nurtures.

Unlike humans, pets love with no strings attached. They love unconditionally and are never judgmental. They don't care how you look, they are enthralled by everything you say, they will always agree, and they are never offended. They will love you, even those times when you know you're unlovable. For the heart patient the unique relationship with a pet may be a necessary first step to recovery. For the hard-driving person some badly needed balance can be given by a pet.

RELIGION AND HEALTH

For many people there is another source of unconditional love more powerful than a pet.

Will praying to God reverse heart disease? I can't make any promises, but I do know that it helps.

I'm a doctor, not a preacher. I would never presume to advise people spiritually. But I do know that people who practice some form of religion enjoy better health. This is based on many studies and from my own observations as a doctor.

In a recent survey of 1,473 people, Kenneth Ferraro, a psychologist at Purdue University, discovered that only 4 percent of regular churchgoers reported ill health, while 9 percent of those who did not had health complaints.[3] While only one-quarter of those who never attended church reported excellent health, 36 percent of those who attended regularly enjoyed excellent health.

The study offered four possible explanations for this preponderance of health in religious people:

- Religious people tend to avoid destructive behaviors like smoking, using drugs, or drinking excessively.

- Religious activity provides a social network for coping and support that is quite different from our secular network.

- Faith gives a special meaning to life and a value system that helps make sense of the world and our lives.

- Religious practice may modify the stress associated with physical suffering and give hope.

THE POWER OF PRAYER

In his excellent book, *Healing Words*, Larry Dossey, M.D., writes how astonished he was to find more than one hundred published studies—using good science—of which "over half showed that prayer brings about significant changes in a variety of living beings."[4] The book documents the far-reaching power of prayer. Dr. Dossey reports that any form of prayer, regardless of faith, is beneficial. After reading his book, you'll wonder why the medical profession has so persistently ignored this source of healing. I know it sounds strange, but the data is powerful. Had a new drug yielded the same results, it would have been heralded as a therapeutic breakthrough and rushed into service.

Why does prayer work? Belivers think they know the reason. For unbelievers all I can suggest is that there are sound psychological reasons for thinking that faith and hope and the feeling of being loved are good for people.

There's much to be said for the powers of the mind healing the body. Mind and body are tightly integrated. Before the word "stress" was popular, doctors wondered just how big its role was in disease. Today we know that much as fleeting thoughts can flush the face, so too negative thoughts can stop bodily functions and create disease. That's stress. And we know that it affects the production of pancreatic enzymes, intestinal peristalsis, and blood flow just by rearing its ugly head.

RELIGION AND BALANCE

I am a Christian and regularly attend the Irvine United Church of Christ. My pastor, Fred Plummer, believes that regular religious activity provides out increasingly complicated lives with a much-needed source of balance. Interestingly, the ancient Arabic definition for the word "religion" is balance. Religion can provide a balance between the inner and outer worlds.

Religion also instills values that make sense. In this materialistic world, it places great importance on such virtues as honesty, responsibility, compassion, loyalty, and friendship. And religion gives you a larger perspective on life. Compared with the sacrifice that Christ made on the cross, giving up bacon and eggs for breakfast shouldn't be such a big deal.

CHAPTER TWENTY-EIGHT

Health and Healing

Agelaus was kind to Acestorides,
  who, if he had lived, would have been lame.
Agelaus decided to operate.

—Nikarchos

Nikarchos, an ancient Roman poet, was having a little fun at the expense of Roman surgeons. But in every satire there is an element of truth. Even back in the days of ancient Rome, patients were scared into unnecessary and dangerous surgery. After two thousand years and countless technological advances you'd think things would have changed. In a lot of ways they have. But in a lot of ways they have not.

MEDICINE, PROGRESS, AND PROBLEMS

Since Nikarchos's time, medicine has made enormous progress, most of it occurring quite recently, at least in historical terms. What we call modern medicine was invented in the past hundred years. And new technologies continue rapidly to transform medicine.

We have all benefited enormously from these changes; they have made life safer, longer, and in many ways healthier. In advanced countries we no longer have to worry about many deadly diseases. We have learned how to treat trauma that once was considered fatal. Infant mortality is way down, life expectancy is way up.

Yet, at the same time, a million Americans die from a treatable, reversible, even avoidable disease. That disease is, to a large extent, the result of our modern life. And the treatments that technology offers us—bypass surgery, cardiac catheterization, even heart transplants—are problematic at best. Technology can solve problems. But it creates new problems as well.

TECHNOLOGY, FRIEND AND FOE

Our modern food industry is a good example of the double-edged nature of technological development. We now can grow and harvest enough food to feed the entire world. The only problem is that much of that food isn't good for us.

In America there is an abundance of food, perhaps too much. We have the most ingenious and productive food industry in the world. The only real obstacle to adequate food consumption is poverty, but that's another problem. Yet, as a nation, we are severely malnourished. I believe that many of the physical, psychological, and social problems we see today are the result of malnutrition.

Technology gives, and technology taketh away. The food industry that gives us ripe fruits and vegetables throughout all four seasons of the year is the same food industry that refines wholesome wheat, discarding the nutritious germ and shell, and leaves us with white flour denuded of all its natural taste and goodness.

And that's just one example.

The marvels of industrial production and high technology have made it possible for most of us to avoid manual labor. And so many of us live a sedentary lifestyle, without enough exercise.

Through the development of architecture, heating, and air conditioning, we have solved the problem of shelter, and we are now able to live in harsh climates and even in previously uninhabitable places. As a result, many of us stay indoors all day and don't get enough fresh air or sunshine.

The automobile gives us mobility undreamed of by previous generations. And so we drive everywhere, get little exercise, and pollute our atmosphere. We never give ourselves a chance to stop and smell the roses.

YOU WANT A REVOLUTION?

While the word is overused, the changes brought about by science and technology over the past three hundred years are, in fact, revolutionary. They have drastically and irrevocably changed almost every aspect of our individual and common lives, for good and for ill. Nor is there any use in wishing they hadn't occurred—these changes were both necessary and inevitable.

The same culture of science and technology that brought us all this essential yet debilitating progress also gave us heart surgery. While heart surgery has undoubtedly saved the lives of many, it has also caused unnecessary pain, suffering, and even death.

NO QUICK FIX

Most heart doctors look at the body as if it were a machine. When the machine is broken they fix it. They never think of treating the root causes of the disease. And they are infatuated with the machines that they use.

The reason so many doctors recommend heart surgery is that it allows them to act in response to a problem. They have been trained to act, and feel frustrated when they can't. That's the main reason they're so disappointed, even angry, when a patient refuses to submit to surgery.

Most doctors are in love with their technology. Too many don't see how it alienates them from their patients.

In days gone by, a doctor would simply talk to the patient and try to find out what was wrong through conversation. Then simple diagnostic tools were developed, like the stethoscope, which allowed the doctor to listen more closely to the patient's body, while still being in personal contact with him. Now medical decisions are being made by professional specialists, some of whom never meet the patient in the flesh. Instead they look at an X ray or examine a tissue sample. The patient is no longer a human being, he's a specimen.

Medical technology can alienate a doctor from his patient. That's one reason there are so many malpractice suits these days. The doctor-patient relationship has degenerated to such an extent that the doctor has become just another service technician. And if the outcome is unsatisfactory, then he must have made a mistake. Back when doctors and patients used to know and trust each other, there was no need for adjudication. If a patient died, his family went to church to pray for his soul.

Now they go to court and sue the doctor.

Not only can medical technology alienate the doctor from the patient, it alienates the patient from himself. In the age of high-tech medicine, the patient is no longer responsible for his own health; he turns that over to the experts. As our life becomes more and more removed from nature, we try increasingly to remedy the disruption with even more unatural measures. In the end we exist only in a world of our own technological creations, and that is a sterile and lonely place.

AN ALTERNATIVE

I reject the mechanical model of medicine. You are a human being, not a machine. Your body is more complex, more unique, and ultimately more awe-inspiring than anything that man could ever manufacture. Your body can even heal itself. If you give it a chance.

My entire professional career has been devoted to healing, not to fixing. My patients come to me because they want something more than a mechanical adjustment. They want to change their lives.

My program may sound radical, but in fact it's rather old-fashioned. I believe in maintaining the body's health by simple, noninvasive means. I hope by now we are sophisticated enough to value simplicity. Yes, we have the technology to rebuild coronary arteries. But is that the right way to cure an ailing heart?

Instead of cutting people open and transplanting their veins, doctors should be helping people to learn to live better and get healthy themselves. The emphasis in medicine needs to change from intervention to care, from fixing to healing, from prescription to teaching, from dictation to discussion, from surgery to therapy. Doctors should treat their patients with respect and with kindness, working with them in a partnership rather than an atmosphere of mutual distrust and hostility. And they should question the necessity of each invasive procedure, especially when those procedures are of dubious benefit or could endanger the patient.

I hope this book has provided you with an alternative to bad medicine. By following the Whitaker Wellness Program you can have a longer, healthier, and happier life. You can take command of your own health, and you can avoid the heart surgery trap.

Where to Find What You Need

American College for Advancement in Medicine (ACAM)
PO Box 3427
Laguna Hills, CA 92653
(714) 583-7666

ACAM is an association of doctors who practice nutritional and preventive medicine, including chelation therapy. For a national roster of ACAM doctors and a pamphlet describing chelation therapy, write to the address above and include two first class stamps for postage.

Healthy Directions, Inc.
P.O. Box 6000
Kearneysville, WV 25430
(800) 722-8008

Healthy Directions is a mail-order source of vitamins and nutritional supplements.

Health & Healing

My monthly newsletter, *Health & Healing*, covers diverse health-related topics. My goal is to keep you abreast of proven alternatives to dangerous medical procedures and drugs, information which you probably won't get from your doctor or the press. I discuss the effectiveness of common treatments and medications, expose what doesn't work, and offer safe, proven alternatives.

Readers of this book can get a one-year subscription at the introductory discount price of $39.95, which is a 42% savings off the regular rate. And I will send you a free bonus copy of my report, "129 Forbidden Medical Secrets and Cures."

To order your subscription, call toll-free (800) 777-5005 and ask for offer #END710, or write

Phillips Publishing
7811 Montrose Road
Potomac, MD 20854

Recipes from the Whitaker Wellness Institute

Features more than 300 recipes for healing meals that meet the dietary guidelines outlined earlier in chapters 13-17. Developed by our gourmet nutritionist, these recipes are used at the Whitaker Wellness Institute every day.

To order your copy at $29.95 (plus shipping and handling) call toll-free 800-705-5559 and ask for offer #BBD28, or write

Phillips Publishing
7811 Montrose Road
Potomac, MD 20854

The Whitaker Wellness Institute

The mainstay of my medical practice is a six-day residential program of evaluation, treatment, education, and motivation at the Whitaker Wellness Institute.

Since its inception in 1979, over 13,000 patients with heart disease, atherosclerosis, high blood pressure, obesity, diabetes, arthritis, and other degenerative diseases have successfully gone through this program.

At Whitaker Wellness, we take a team approach to help each individual patient. Education is high on the list. If you are striving for improved or optimum health, you need a game plan. In brief the program includes:

- Complete medical assessment with emphasis on the cardiovascular system.

- Seminars on the nature of our modern day diseases, the best approach for treating them, and the pitfalls of modern aggressive techniques.

- Implementation of an individual exercise program, and a seminar on the effects of exercise.

- Explanation of the role of nutritional supplements, and why they are necessary for modern life and optimal health.

- Classes in food preparation, shopping, and eating in restaurants. Guidelines for healthy living, not dieting.

Patients stay at a class A resort hotel across the street from my office in Newport Beach, California. Most of the week's activities take place in the hotel. Low-fat, high complex carbohydrate meals, including meals from *Recipes from the Whitaker Wellness Institute,* are catered by our gourmet chef.

The majority of the week's medical expenses are covered by most insurance plans and Medicare, and we encourage the participation of spouses for a minimal fee to cover the cost of meals. They are invited to attend all of the lectures and activities. For more information, please contact my office:

Whitaker Wellness Institute
4321 Birch Street, Suite 100
Newport Bearch, CA 92660
(714) 851-1550 (phone)
(714) 851-9970 (fax)

NOTES

CHAPTER 2

1. David Brown, "Fixing Hearts and Other Rewards of Specialists: Doctors Build Careers Without Burden of Treating 'Whole' Patient," *Washington Post,* 7 November 1993.

2. The Veterans Administration Coronary Artery Bypass Surgery Cooperative Study Group, "Eleven Year Survival in the Veterans Administration Randomized Trial of Coronary Bypass Surgery for Stable Angina," *New England Journal of Medicine* 311 (1984): 1333-1339.

3. Marvin L. Murphy, et al., "Treatment of Chronic Stable Angina: A Preliminary Report of Survival Data of the Randomized Veterans Administration Cooperative Study," *New England Journal of Medicine* 297 (1977): 621-627.

4. Coronary Artery Surgery Study (CASS), "A Randomized Trial of Coronary Artery Bypass Surgery: Quality of Life in Patients Randomly Assigned to Treatment Groups," *Circulation* 68, no. 5 (1983): 951-960.

5. W. J. Rogers, et al., "Ten year follow-up of quality of life in patients randomized to receive medical therapy or coronary artery bypass grafts and surgery. The Coronary Artery: Surgery Study," *Circulation* 82, no. 5 (November 1990): 1859-1862.

6. Associated Press, "Many Men with Angina Don't Need Bypass Surgery," *New York Times,* 20 November 1990.

7. G. V. R. K. Sharma, et al., "Identification of Unstable Angina Patients Who Have Favorable Outcome with Medical or Surgical Therapy (Eight-Year Follow-up of the Veterans Administration Cooperative Study)," *American Journal of Cardiology* 74 (September 1, 1994): 454-458.

8. Mark McClellan, et al., "Does More Intensive Treatment of Acute Myocardial Infarction in the Elderly Reduce Mortality? Analysis Using Instrumental Variables," *Journal of American Medical Association* 272, no. 11 (September 21, 1995): 859-866.

9. Edvardas Varnauskas, et al., "Twelve Year Follow-Up of Survival in the Randomized European Coronary Surgery Study," *New England Journal of Medicine* 319 (August 11, 1988): 332-337.

10. Harvey B. Simon, *Conquering Heart Disease* (Boston: Little Brown, 1994), 396.

11. Cashen, W. Linda, et al., "Accelerated Progression of Atherosclerosis in Coronary Vessels with Minimal Lesions that Are Bypassed," *New England Journal of Medicine* 311 (September 27, 1984): 824-828.

12. Nicholas L. Depace, M.D. and Steven K. Darinsky, M.D., "Prevention of

further atherosclerosis in Coronary Artery Bypass Graft patients," *Cardiac and Non-Cardiac Complications of Open Heart Surgery: Prevention, Diagnosis, and Treatment* (New York: Futura Publishing, 1992).

13. Both Rand and AHA stats from Judy Foreman, "Heart Bypass May Disrupt Thinking," *Boston Globe*, 8 February 1993.

14. David Harris, et al., "Brain Swelling in First Hour After Coronary Artery Bypass Surgery," *Lancet* 342 (September 4, 1993): 586-587.

15. Jeff Goldberg, "Heart Surgery's Hidden Heartbreak," *Omni*, November 1992.

16. Gina Kolata, "Theory May Explain Mystery of Deaths After Heart Bypass," *New York Times*, 18 December 1990.

17. Constance Monroe Winsow, et al., "The Appropriateness of Performing Coronary Artery Bypass Surgery," *Journal of the American Medical Association* 260, no. 4 (July 22/29, 1988).

CHAPTER 3

1. P. H. Podrid, T. B. Graboys, and B. Lown, "Prognosis of Medically Treated Patients with Coronary Artery Disease with Profound ST-Segment Depression During Exercise Testing," *New England Journal of Medicine* 305 (November 5, 1981): 1111-1116.

2. W. Hueb, et al., "Two to Eight Year Survival Rates in Patients Who Refused Coronary Artery Bypass Grafting," *American Journal of Cardiology* 63, no. 3 (January 1989): 155-159.

3. Nicholas Danchin, "Ten-year Follow-up of Patients with Single Vessel Coronary Artery Disease that Was Suitable for Percutaneous Transluminal Coronary Angioplasty," *British Heart Journal* 59 (1988): 275-279.

4. Dean Ornish, et al., "Effects of stress management training and dietary training in treating ischemic heart disease," *Journal of the American Medical Association* 249 (1983): 54-59.

5. Thomas B. Graboys, "Results of a Second Opinion Program for Coronary Artery Bypass Graft Surgery," *Journal of the American Medical Association* 258 (1987): 1611-1614.

6. Ibid.

7. Henry McIntosh, M.D., "Second Opinions by Aortocoronary Bypass Grafting are Beneficial," *Journal of the American Medical Association*, (September 25, 1987).

CHAPTER 4

1. National Heart, Lung, and Blood Institute, an investigation of angiogram reliability, presented at the 1979 American Heart Association Meeting, Anaheim, California.

2. Dr. Leonard M. Zir, "Interobserver Variability in Coronary Angiography," *Circulation* 53, no. 4 (April 1976): 627-632.

3. Carl W. White, M.D., et al., "Does Visual Interpretation of the Coronary Arteriogram Predict the Physiologic Importance of Coronary Stenosis?" *New England Journal of Medicine* 310, no. 13 (March 29, 1984): 819-824.

4. T. B. Graboys, et al., "Results of a second-opinion trial among patients recommended for coronary angiography," *Journal of the American Medical Association* 268, no. 18 (November 11, 1992): 2537-2540.

CHAPTER 5

1. Peter Aleshire, "The Dangers of Friendly Fire," *Arizona Republic,* 18 February 1990.

2. Dr. Andreas Greuntzig, et al., "Non-operative Dilation of Coronary Artery Stenosis: Percutaneous Transluminal Coronary Angioplasty," *New England Journal of Medicine* 301, no. 2 (July 12): 61-68.

3. Letter to the Editor, "The Spoof Factor," *Journal of American College of Cardiology* 14 (1989): 125.

4. Sabrice S. Larrazet, M.D., et al., "Angioscopy after Laser and Balloon Coronary Angioplasty," *Journal of American College of Cardiology* 23, no.6 (May 1994).

5. Charles D. Bankhead, "Restenosis," *Medical World News* (February 1991): 26-34.

6. Mauro Moscucci, et al., "Peripheral Vascular Complications of Directional Coronary Atherectomy and Stenting: Predictors, Management, and Outcome," *American Journal of Cardiology* 74 (September 1, 1994): 448-453.

7. Eric J. Topol, "A compassion of directional atherectomy with coronary angioplasty in patients with coronary artery disease," *New England Journal of Medicine* 329, no. 4 (July 22, 1993): 221-227.

8. Quoted in Tim Friend, "Drug Therapy can be as Helpful as Angioplasty," *USA Today,* 15 November 1994.

9. S. B. King, et al., "A randomized trial comparing coronary angioplasty with coronary bypass surgery," *New England Journal of Medicine* 331, no. 16 (October 20, 1994): 1044-1050. C. W. Hamm, et al., "A Randomized study of coronary angioplasty compared with bypass surgery in patients with symptomatic multivessel coronary disease," *New England Journal of Medicine* 331, no. 16 (October 20, 1994): 1038-1043.

CHAPTER 6

1. "Heart Surgery Study Finds Risk is Greater for Women," *Wall Street Journal,* 19 March 1991, p. B3.

2. Quoted in Gina Kolata, "Study Finds Bias in Way Women Are Evaluated for Heart Bypass," *The New York Times,* 16 April 1990, p. A15.

3. Cited in Judy Foreman, "Angioplasty risks found for women," *Boston Globe,* 9 March 1993, p. 1.

4. Ibid.

5. Ibid.

6. Cited in Robin Herman, "Too Much Heart Surgery? Doctors Debate Role of Diagnostic Test," *The Washington Post*, 17 November 1992, p. Z8.

CHAPTER 7

1. Eugene Braunwald, "Coronary Artery Surgery at the Crossroads," *New England Journal of Medicine* 297, no. 12 (September 22, 1977): 661-663.

2. American Heart Association, 1994 statistical fact sheet.

3. Ibid.

4. Herman C. B. Denber, "Biological and Psychological Implications," *Futura* (Armonic, New York, 1995), 38.

5. "The Cardiac Money Machine," *Consumer Reports*, July 1992.

6. Ibid.

7. Ibid.

8. Ibid.

9. Ibid.

CHAPTER 10

1. Julian Whitaker, M.D., *Health & Healing*, May 1992, Phillips Publishing, Potomac, MD.

2. Ibid.

CHAPTER 11

1. Valek, J., et al., "Serum linoleic acid and cardiovascular death in postin-farction middle-aged men," *Athersclerosis* 54 (1885):11-18. Wood, D.A. et al., "Adipose tissue and platelet fatty acids and coronary heart disease in Scottish men," *Lancet* (July 21, 1984): 117-121. Simpson H. et al., "Low dietary intake of linoleic acid predisposes to myocardial infarction," *Br Medical Journal* 285(1982): 684.

CHAPTER 12

1. Julian Whitaker, M.D., *Health & Healing*, March 1993, Phillips Publishing, Potomac, MD.

CHAPTER 19

1. M. J. Stampfer, et al., "Vitamin consumption and the risk of coronary disease in women," *New England Journal of Medicine* 328 (May 20, 1993): 1444-1449.

CHAPTER 20

1. P. Menasche, C. Grousset, et al., "A promising approach for improving the recovery of heart transplants: Prevention of free radical injury through iron chelation by deferoxamine," *Journal of Thoracic and Cardio Surgery* 100 (July 1990): 13-21.

CHAPTER 22

1. T. Kamikawa, et al., "Effects of coenzyme Q10 on exercise tolerance in chronic stable angina," *American Journal of Cardiology* 56 (1985): 247-251.

2. P.H. Langsjoen, et al., "Long-term efficacy and safety of coenzyme Q10 therapy for idiopathic dilated cardiomyopathy," *American Journal of Cardiology*, 65 (1990): 521-523.

3. Richard Quinn, *Left for Dead*, (Minnestoa: R.F. Quinn Publishers, 1992).

CHAPTER 23

1. F. Batmanghelidj, M.D., *Your Body's Many Cries for Water*, (Falls Church, VA: Global Health Solutions, Inc., 1992).

CHAPTER 24

1. *Medical Regimens: Causes of Non-Compliance*. Washington D.C.: Office of Inspector General, Dept. of Health and Human Services, June 1990.

2. Food and Drug Administration, *A National Survey of Prescription Drug Information Provided to Patients* (1986).

3. Editorial, "Beware the Risks in Prescription Drugs." *USA Today*, 28 July 1994.

4. Quoted in "Reduce risks in prescription drugs," *USA Today*, 1 September 1994, p. A8.

5. Dr. Dean Ornish, et al., "Can lifestyle changes reverse coronary artery disease?" *Lancet* 336 (1990): 129-133.

CHAPTER 25

1. Professor Jeremy N. Morris, "Coronary heart disease and physical activity of work," *Lancet* (Nov. 21 and Nov. 28, 1953).

2. Professor Jeremy N. Morris, "Vigorous Exercise in Leisure Time in the Incidence of Coronary Heart Disease," *Lancet* (17 February 1973): 333-339.

3. Dieter M. Kramsch, "Reduction of Coronary Athersclerosis by Moderate Conditioning Exercise in Monkeys on an Atherogenic Diet," *New England Journal of Medicine* 305 (December 1981): 1483-1489.

4. M. A. Fiatarone, et al., "Exercise training and nutritional supplementation for physical frailty in very elderly people," *New England Journal of Medicine* 330, no. 25 (June 23, 1994): 1769-1775.

CHAPTER 26

1. N. E. Clarke, "Atherosclerosis, occlusive vascular disease and EDTA," *American Journal of Cardiology* 6 (1960): 122-126.

2. E. Olszwerer and J. P. Carter, "EDTA chelation therapy in chronic degenerative disease," *Medical Hypotheses* 27 (1988): 41-49.

3. Ibid.

4. Jane Heimlich, *What your doctor won't tell you* (New York: HarperCollins, 1990), 122.

CHAPTER 27

1. Julian Whitaker, M.D., *Health & Healing*, November 1991, Phillips Publishing, Potomac, MD.

2. Ibid.

3. Kenneth F. Ferraro and C.M. Albrecht-Jensen, "Does religion influence health?" *J. Scientific Study Religion* 30 (1991): 193-20

4. Larry Dossey, *Healing Words*.

INDEX

ACAM. *See* American College of
Advancement in Medicine
Adenosine triphosphate
  EDTA chelation therapy and, 255
  magnesium and, 203-204
Adrenaline, 223
Aerobic dancing, 240-241
Aggressive-conservative program, 6-7
Alcohol, 155
Allicin, 147
Alpha-linolenic acid, 105-106
ALS. *See* Lou Gehrig's disease
Aluminum, 90, 199
Alzheimer's disease, 84
American College of Advancement in
  Medicine, 40, 253, 269
American College of Cardiology, 22
American Heart Association, 22
Amino acids
  function, 194-195
  sulphur-containing, 88
Anemia, 198
Angina
  beta blockers treatment, 223-225
  calcium channel blockers
    treatment, 224-225
  causes of, 33-34
  coenzyme Q10 and, 198
  as determinant for bypass surgery,
    32
  exercise stress test and, 49
  fats and, 104-105
  magnesium ATP treatment, 203
  nitroglycerin treatment, 221-223,
    224-225
  occurrence after bypass surgery,
    21-22
  omega-3 fatty acids and, 106
  relief following bypass surgery,
    34-35
  vitamin E and, 185
Angiograms
  accuracy of, 45-48

alternatives, 48-51
dangers of, 44-45
description, 43-44
development of, 15
profit margins, 72
usefulness, 51-52
Angioplasty
  cardiologists and, 56, 61-62
  case study, 53-54
  compared with bypass surgery, 60-61
  complications, 9, 57-59
  description, 54
  mortality rate, 54
  profit margins, 72
  side effects, 54-55
Angioscope, 57
Animal foods, 98
Antioxidants
  beta carotene, 183-184
  case study, 7
  fat oxidation prevention, 109
  free radicals and, 88-92
  nutritional supplements and, 177
  vitamin C, 181-183
  vitamin E, 184-187
Anxiety, 23
Apple Raisin Noodle Pudding recipe,
  171
Arginine. *See* L-arginine
Arrhythmia. *See* Cardiac arrhythmia
Arteries
  cholesterol and, 80
  damage from fat in blood, 79
  exercise and, 233-234
  function, 78
  high blood pressure and, 80
  smoking and, 79
  vitamin C deficiency and, 80
Arteriosclerosis, 78
Artery constriction, 25
Artery stenosis, 21
Arthritis
  free radicals and, 84

omega-3 fatty acids and, 106
Ascorbic acid. *See* Vitamin C
Atherectomy, 9, 59-60
Atherosclerosis, 78
ATP. *See* Adenosine triphosphate
Author background, xi-xvi
Avocado, 153

Balloon angioplasty. *See* Angioplasty
Barrett-Connor, Elizabeth, 212
Batmanghelidj, F., 215
Baylor College of Medicine, 15
Beans, 148-149
Beta blockers
  angina treatment, 223-225
  function, 114
Beta carotene
  deficiency symptoms, 184
  function, 88-91
  importance of, 183
  RDA, 184
  sources of, 147
  supplement regimen case study, 7
Bicycling, 238-239
Bile, 107-108
Blocadren, 223
Blockages, 21, 47
Blood cholesterol. *See* Cholesterol
Blood clots. *See* Clotting
Blood pressure. *See* High blood
  pressure
Brain damage, 22-23
Brain swelling, 23
Brassinin, 179
Braunwald, Eugene, 70
Brewer, H. Bryan, 95
Brewer's yeast, 190, 191
Brown rice, 150
Butter, 139-140
Bypass surgery
  as an industry, 69-71
  choosing surgery for the wrong
    reasons, 33-38
  complications, 6
  conflicts of interest, 72-73
  costs of, 8
  death rates, 24
  description, 3-6
  effectiveness of, 15-18

history of, 14-15
insurance and, 72-73
as last option, 26
number of operations performed,
  71
as a placebo, 35
postoperative heart attacks, 24-25
profitability of operations, 71-73
rate of unnecessary operations,
  25-26
reasons for choosing surgery, 29-32
reclosure of grafted veins, 20-22
scare tactics, 9-11, 13-14
second opinions, 39-41
side effects, 22-24

Cabbage, 147
CAD. *See* Coronary artery disease
Cadmium, 7, 90
Calan, 224
Calcium channel blockers
  angina treatment, 224-225
  case study, 7
  compared with magnesium
    supplements, 114, 202, 224
  heart disease and, 119
Calcium deficiencies, 152
Cancer
  beta carotene and, 183
  cholesterol saturation and, 99
  cruciferous vegetables and, 179
  essential fatty acids deficiency and,
    106
  free radicals and, 84, 85
  polyunsaturated fats and, 107
Candidiasis, 195
Canned foods
  beans, 149
  fruits and vegetables, 152
Capillaries, 102-103
Capsaicin, 211
Carbohydrates, 98-99, 134-135
Carbon monoxide, 90
Cardene, 224
Cardiac arrhythmia
blood pressure medication and,
  113-114
  magnesium and, 202-203
Cardiac causalgia, 23-24

Cardiac risk checklist, 39-40
Cardiologists
  angioplasty and, 56, 61-62
  profitability of bypass surgeries and,
    71-73
Cardiomyopathy
  case study, 205-206
  coenzyme Q10 and, 198
Cardizem, 224
Carnitine. *See* L-carnitine
Case studies
  angioplasty, 53-54
  antioxidants, 7
  beta carotene, 7
  calcium channel blockers, 7
  L-carnitine, 7, 206
  coenzyme Q10, 7, 206
  L-dopa, 206
  drug therapy, 7
  EDTA chelation therapy, 7, 252-253
  exercise, 7
  free radicals, 7
  low-fat diet, 7
  magnesium supplement regimen, 7
  nitroglycerin, 7
  nutritional supplements, 7
  vitamin C supplement regimen, 7
  vitamin E, 7, 184-185
  Whitaker Wellness Institute, 120-126
CASS. *See* Coronary Artery Surgery
  Study
Cataracts, 183
Cayenne pepper, 210-211
Celiac disease, 150
Chest pain. *See* Angina
Chicken Kabobs recipe, 168
Chili recipe, 164
Chlorine, 90
Cholesterol
  alcohol and, 155
  arterial damage, 80
  blood pressure medication and,
    113-114
  effect of heat and oxygen, 100
  exercise and, 233
  free radicals and, 87, 100
  functions, 94
  lipoproteins, 94-95
  manufactured in the body, 93

meats and, 152
  omega-3 fatty acids and, 106
  safe levels for blood cholesterol, 97
  saturation, 99
  sources of, 98
  vitamin C and, 96-97
Cholesterol saturation, 99
Chromium, 191
Chylomicrons, 103
Clarke, Norman, 249
Clotting
  high blood pressure and, 112
  vitamin E and, 185
Coenzyme Q10
  case studies, 7, 206
  heart disease and, 207
  importance of, 197-198
Cognitive function, 22
Collateral arteries, 234
Complex carbohydrates, 134-135
Conflicts of interest, 72-73
Congestive heart failure
  calcium channel blockers and, 224
  high blood pressure and, 112
Contraindications, 219
Cooke, John P., 209
Copper, 88, 90, 191
CoQ10. *See* Coenzyme Q10
Corgard, 223
Corn, 149-150
Corn Bread recipe, 162
Coronary artery disease, 36-37
Coronary artery spasms, 33-34
Coronary Artery Surgery Study
  follow-up of second study, 18-19
  original study, 17-18
  ten-year follow-up study, 18
Cruciferous vegetables, 147, 179
Cysteine. *See* L-cysteine

D-alpha tocopherol, 185, 186
Danchin, Nicholas, 37-38
Degassing beans, 148
Depression
  blood pressure medication and, 114
  bypass surgery and, 23
  overview, 257-258
  pets and, 258-260
  religion and health, 260-262

DHEA, 211-213
Diabetes
  essential fatty acids deficiency and,
    106
  L-arginine and, 210
  L-cysteine and, 195
Diastolic pressure, 112
Diet
  comparing Western and Oriental
diets, 132-133
  four pillars of therapy, 119-120
  lowering high blood pressure and,
    115-116
  making changes, 131
Diet plan
  beans, 148-149
  brown rice compared with other
    grains, 150
  corn, 149-150
  foods to avoid, 156-159
  foods to eat sparingly, 152-156
  fresh fruits, 146
  fresh vegetables, 146-147
  frozen fruits and vegetables, 147-
    148
  grains, 151
  guidelines, 145-146, 160
  potatoes, 149
Digestive enzymes, 197
Directional atherectomy, 59-60
Diuretics, 113-114, 217
DNA, 85
Dopamine, 208, 258
Dossey, Larry, 261
Drug therapy
  beta blockers, 223-225
  calcium channel blockers, 224-225
  case study, 7
  as catalyst for free radicals, 90
  heart disease and, 119-120
  nitroglycerin, 221-223, 224-225
  risks of, 220
  wellness therapy and, 225

Eastern diets, 98-99
Echocardiography, 50
Eczema, 106
Edema, 159
EDRF. *See* Endothelium-derived

relaxing factor
EDTA chelation therapy
  benefits of, 247-248
  case studies, 7, 252-253
  description of procedure, 254-255
  history of, 248-250
  how it works, 250-251
  maintenance, 256
  other therapies and, 255
  overview, 119-120
  problems of, 253-254
  safety, 251
Egg substitutes, 158-159
Eggs, 98, 155
Ejection fraction, 31-32, 50-51
EKG. *See* Electrocardiogram
Electrocardiogram, 48-49
Emergency bypass surgery, 54, 61
Endorphins, 231
Endothelium-derived relaxing factor,
  209
Enzymes, 91, 197
Epinephrine, 231
Essential fatty acids, 105-106, 196
Essential minerals, 191-194
Ethylene diamine tetracidic acid. *See*
  EDTA chelation therapy
EuroCASS. *See* European Coronary
  Artery Surgery Study
European Coronary Artery Surgery
  Study, 19-20
Exercise
  aerobic dancing, 240-241
  benefits from, 119-120, 229
  case study, 7
  choosing an exercise, 236-237
  consulting a doctor, 235
  effect on the heart, 232-234
  enjoying exercise, 243
  jogging, 238
  lowering high blood pressure and,
    115
  reasons for, 230-231
  road bicycling, 239
  stationary bicycling, 238-239
  stretching, 241
  swimming, 239-240
  walking, 237
  weight training, 241-242

work-related, 231-232
Exercise stress test, 35-36, 49, 235

Fat imbalance, 113
Fatigue, 114
Fats
  angina and, 104-105
  arterial damage and, 79
  butter and margarine, 139-140
  calculating percentage of fat, 136-137
  essential, 105-106, 196
  free radicals and, 87-88
  oxidation of, 109
  oxygen supply and, 101-103
  recommended intake, 110
  saturated, 107-108
  triglycerides, 108
  unsaturated, 107
Favaloro, Rene, 15
Ferraro, Kenneth, 260
Fiber, 107-108, 146
Fiberless sugars, 156-157
Fibrinolysis, 233
Fish, 154
Fish oil, 143
Flax oil, 142-143, 196
Flesh foods, 98
Flour, 151
Fluoride, 90
Folic acid, 195
Folkers, Karl, 207
Food and Drug Administration, 176, 211, 213, 251
Food industry, 264-265
Four pillars of therapy, 119-126
Free radicals
  antioxidants and, 88-92
  case study, 7
  catalysts, 90
  chemical process, 84-85
  development of, 85-86
  diet and, 91-92
  fats and, 87-88
  heart disease and, 86-87
  importance of, 83-84
  vitamin C and, 182
Fresh fruits, 146
Fresh vegetables, 146-147

Frozen fruits and vegetables, 147-148
Frozen yogurt, 156, 158
Fructose, 153
Fruit Crisp recipe, 172
Fruit juices, 153
Fruits, 146

Gallstones, 107
Ginkgo biloba, 197
Glucose-6-phosphate dehydrogenase, 212
Glutathione, 90
Gluten intolerance, 150
Gout, 193-194
Graboys, Thomas, 39
Grains, 150-151
Green vegetables, 146-147
Greuntzig, Andreas R., 55
Ground meats, 157

Hallucinations, 23
Hand-eye coordination, 23
Harvard Medical School, 20
HDL. *See* High-density lipoproteins
Headaches, 221
Healing Words, 261
Health & Healing, 270
Healthy Directions, Inc., 269-270
Heart attacks
  blood pressure medication and, 113-114
  as bypass surgery side effect, 23, 24-25
  calcium channel blockers and, 224
  magnesium survival and, 202
Heart disease
  arterial damage and, 79-80
  beta carotene and, 183
  in bypassed arteries, 20-22
  cardiac arrhythmia and, 202-203
  description, 77-78
  essential fatty acids deficiency and, 106
  free radicals and, 86-87
  high blood pressure and, 112
  incidence of, xi
  magnesium supplements and, 192
  meats and, 152
  mortality rate, 71

plaque development, 80
silent development of, 81-82
Heart Foods, 210
Heart-lung machine
development of, 15
microemboli and, 23
use in bypass surgery, 4-6
Heart medication, 7
Heart surgery
alternative to, 267-268
medical technology and, 266-267
Heavy metals, 7
Hemorrhage, 23
Hexavalent chromium, 90
High blood pressure
arterial damage, 80
causes of, 113
description, 111-112
magnesium and, 201-202
medication problems, 113-114
omega-3 fatty acids and, 106
safe methods of lowering, 115
as a treatable condition, 112
High-density lipoproteins
alcohol and, 155
chromium and, 191
compared with LDL, 94-96
High-risk patients, 18-19
Holter monitoring, 49
Hormones, 211-213
Hydrogenation, 140
Hypertension, 185
Hypotension, 224

Iatrogenesis, 54
Ice cream, 158
Immune system repression
polyunsaturated fats and, 107
saturated fats and, 108
Impotence, 114
Inderal, 223
Insoluble fiber, 146
Intermittent claudication
EDTA chelation therapy, 250
vitamin E and, 185
Interobserver variability, 45-46
Iron, 198
Irregular heartbeat
as bypass surgery side effect, 24

potassium supplements and, 192
Ischemic heart disease
EDTA chelation therapy, 250
vitamin E and, 185
Isoptin, 224
Isositol hexaniacinate, 190
Isothiocyanates, 179

Japanese diets, 98-99, 132-133
Jogging, 238
Johnson, Dudley, 15
Juices, 153

Kempner, Walter, 116
Kidney disease, 112
Kidney failure
magnesium ATP treatment, 203
magnesium supplements and, 192
Kidney stones
L-cysteine and, 195

L-arginine, 208-210
L-carnitine
case studies, 7, 206
function, 195
heart disease and, 207-208
L-cysteine, 88, 91, 195
L-dopa, 190
case study, 206
heart disease and, 208
Lasagna Florentine recipe, 165-166
LDL. *See* Low-density lipoproteins
Lead, 7, 90
Left for Dead, 210
Left main coronary artery, 30-31
Left ventricle, 32
Lentil Stew recipe, 163
Lentils, 149
Lifestyle
high blood pressure and, 113
program for change, 11-12
Lignans, 143
Linoleic acid, 105-106
Linolenic acid, 105-106
Linseed oil, 196
Lipid peroxides, 87-88
Lipoproteins, 94
Liver, 95
Liver failure, 203

LNA. *See* Alpha-linolenic acid
Lopressor, 223
Lou Gehrig's disease, 84
Low-density lipoproteins
  compared with HDL, 94-96
  free radicals and, 100
  margarine and, 140
  vitamin E and, 184
Low-fat diet
  case study, 7
  lowering high blood pressure and,
    115-116
Low-risk patients, 18-19
Lown Cardiovascular Center, 39
Lown group
  cardiac risk checklist, 39-40
  ST-segment depression study, 36
Lysine, 195

Magnesium
  benefits of, 192
  blood pressure medication and,
    113-114
  blood pressure reduction, 201-202
  cardiac arrhythmia and, 202-203
  compared with calcium channel
    blockers, 224
  fresh vegetables and, 146-147
  heart attack survival and, 202
  high-energy magnesium, 203-204
  importance of, 201
  L-cysteine and, 195
  lowering high blood pressure and,
    115-116
  suggestions, 204
  supplement regimen case study, 7
Magnesium ATP, 203-204
Magnesium gluconate, 192
Mammary artery, 15
Manganese, 88, 193
Margarine, 158-159
Maximum heart rate, 235
Mayonnaise, 142, 157
Meats, 152, 156
Medicaid, 72
Medical profession, xi-xii
Medical therapy
  advances in, 263-264
  compared with heart surgery

  results, 16-20
  heart disease and, 119-120
  severe coronary artery disease and,
    36-37
Menopause, 66
Mercury, 7, 90
Methionine, 195
Microemboli, 23
Molybdenum, 193-194
Monounsaturated fats, 107
Morris, Jeremy, 231-232
Mortality rates
  angioplasty, 54
  bypass surgery, 24
  bypass surgery for women, 63-64
  CASS study, 17
  heart disease, 71
  VACS study, 16
MSG, 195
Multiple bypass surgery. *See* Bypass
surgery
Murkin, John, 23

National Heart, Lung, and Blood
  Institute, 45
Natural bypass, 234
Natural foods, 133-134
Neurobehavioral defects, 22
Neurotransmitters, 194-195
Niacin, 189-190
Nitrates, 90, 156
Nitric oxide, 209
Nitrites, 90
Nitroglycerin
  angina treatment, 221-223, 224-225
  case study, 7
  heart disease and, 119
  nitric oxide and, 209
NO. *See* Nitric oxide
Nonfat milk, 153-154
Nonfat yogurt, 155-156
Noninvasive tests, 48-51
Nonsurgical program, 11-12
Noradrenaline, 231
Normodyne, 223
Northern New England Cardiovascu-
  lar Study Group, 63-64
Nut butters, 158
Nutrient deficiency

high blood pressure and, 113
stages of, 176-177
Nutritional supplements
aluminum and, 199
amino acids, 194-195
B vitamins, 189-190
case study, 7
coenzyme, 197-198
enzymes, 197
essential fatty acids, 196
essential minerals, 191-194
ginkgo biloba, 197
how to take, 177-178
iron and, 198
necessity of, 119-120, 175
nutrient deficiency, 176-177
RDAs and, 176
stockpiling nutrients, 177
whole foods diet and, 178-179
Nuts, 156

Oils, 141, 157
Oily vitamins, 186
Oleic acid, 142
Olive oil, 142, 154
Omega-3 fatty acids, 105-106, 110,
142-143
Omega-6 fatty acids, 105, 142-143
Omelet recipe, 170
"129 Forbidden Medical Secrets and
Cures," 270
Organ meats, 98
Oriental diets, 98-99, 132-133
Ornish, Dean, 225
Oxidation, 84, 88

Parkinson's disease, 208
Pauling, Linus, 96
Peanut butter, 158
Percutaneous transluminal coronary
angioplasty. *See* Angioplasty
Perioperative death
bypass surgery and, 6
CASS study, 17
of repeat bypass patients, 24
VACS study, 16
Peripheral vascular disease, 250
Pesticides, 147

PET scan. *See* Positron emission
tomography
Pet therapy, 258-260
Phenethyl isothiocyanates, 179
Phospholipids, 95
Phytochemicals, 178-179
Plaque
in bypassed arteries, 21
free radicals and, 86-87
Pneumonia, 23
Polynuclear aromatic hydrocarbons,
90
Polyunsaturated fats, 107
Pork, 156
Positron emission tomography, 50
Potassium
benefits of, 192-193
blood pressure medication and,
113-114
lowering high blood pressure and,
115-116
sodium and, 159
Potatoes, 149
Poultry, 154, 156
Prayer, 261-262
Prescription drugs. *See also* Drug
therapy
as catalysts for free radicals, 90
contraindications, 219
high blood pressure and, 113-114
risks of, 220
Prinzmetal's variant angina, 34
Pritikin, Nathan, xiv-xv
Procardia, 224
Processed foods, 133-134, 156
Progressive exercise. *See* Exercise
Prostaglandins
free radicals and, 87
zinc and, 191
Protein
reducing amount in diet, 135-136
from vegetarian diets, 151
Protein flag, 96-97
Psoriasis, 106
PTCA. *See* Angioplasty
Pyridoxine, 190
Quinn, Richard, 210

Radiation, 88
Rand Corporation, 22, 25-26
Rath, Matthias, 96
RDAs. *See* Recommended Daily
Allowances
*Recipes from the Whitaker Wellness
Institute*, 160-172, 270
Reclosure. *See* Restenosis
Recommended Daily Allowances
  beta carotene, 184
  heart disease and, 176
  vitamin C, 182
Red blood cells, 102
Red meats, 156
Reflexes, 23
Religion, 260-262
Reoperation, 24
Restenosis, 57-58
"Results of a Second-Opinion
  Program for Coronary Artery
  Bypass Graft Surgery," 39
Reversing Heart Disease, 124, 126
Rheumatic heart disease, 185
Rib spreader, 4
Rice and fruit diet, 116
Rice Raffaele recipe, 167
Road bicycling, 239
Roasted nuts, 158
Rotational atherectomy, 59-60
Rule of nine, 136-137

Salt, 113, 159
Saturated fats
  foods with high contents, 141
  meats and, 152
  problems from, 107-108
Scar tissue, 185
Scare tactics, 9-11, 13-14
Second opinions, 39-41
Sectral, 223
Seeds, 156
Selenium, 88, 91, 194
Serotonin, 258
Sesame Chicken Kabobs recipe, 168
Short-term memory, 23
Single-vessel disease, 37-38
Singlet oxygen, 89-90
Skim milk, 153-154
Skinless poultry, 154

Skipping heart. *See* Cardiac arrhythmia
Smoking, 79
Sodium, 159
Sodium molybdate, 194
Sodium:potassium ratio, 115
Soluble fiber, 146
Spicy Chili recipe, 164
Sprue disease, 150
ST-segment depression, 35-36
Stable angina, 34
Starches, 134-135
Stationary bicycling, 238-239
Stent, 58-59
Stress test. *See* Exercise stress test;
  Thallium stress test
Stretching, 241
Stroke
  blood clots and, 112
  bypass surgery and, 22, 23
  high blood pressure and, 112
Sugar intake, 113
Sulforaphane, 179
Sulphur-containing amino acids, 88
Sulphur-containing vegetables, 147
Surgical palliation, 17-18
Swelling, 159
Swimming, 239-240
Synthetic drugs, 90
Systolic pressure, 112

Technology
  advances in medical technology,
    263-264
  food industry, 264-265
  negative aspects of, 265-266
Tenormin, 223
Thallium stress test, 50
Trandate, 223
Triglycerides, 108, 113-114
Triple-vessel disease, 32

Ubiquinone, 197-198
Unsaturated fats, 87-88, 107
Unstable angina, 34
Uric acid
  meats and, 152
  molybdenum supplements and,
    193-194

VACS. *See* Veterans Administration
  Cooperative Study
Vegetable Tostada recipe, 169
Vegetables
  importance of, 146-147
  phytochemicals, 178-179
Vegetarian diet
  heart disease and, 132-133
  protein intake, 151
Ventricular tachycardia, 203
Very low density lipoproteins, 95
Veterans Administration Cooperative
Study, 16-17
Visken, 223
Vitamin A
  beta carotene and, 183
  free radicals and, 88
Vitamin B3, 189-190
Vitamin B6, 190, 195
Vitamin B12
  EDTA chelation therapy and, 255
  L-cysteine and, 195
Vitamin B complex, 7
Vitamin C
  cholesterol and, 96-97
  deficiency and arterial damage, 80
  free radicals and, 88-91
  importance of, 181-182
  RDA, 182
  sources, 183
  supplement regimen case study, 7
  symptoms of deficiency, 182-183
Vitamin deficiency, 176-177
Vitamin E
  case studies, 7, 184-185
  deficiency symptoms, 185
  free radicals and, 88-91
  heart disease and, 184
  topical application, 185
Vitamins, 7
VLDL. *See* Very low density
  lipoproteins

Walking, 237
Water, 159, 215-216
Water pills, 113-114
Weight training, 241-242
Wellness Program, xvi
Western diets, 98-99, 132-133
Western Omelet recipe, 170
Wheat, 150
Whitaker Wellness Institute
  address, 127, 272
  case studies, 120-126
  description, 271-272
  founding of, xv-xvi
  four pillars of therapy, 119
  phone number, 127
  recipes, 161-172, 270-271
Whole foods, 133-134
Whole grain flours, 153
Wilson's disease, 191
Women
  angiograms and, 64-65
  angioplasty and, 65
  bypass surgery and, 63-64
  mortality rate from bypass surgery,
    63-64
  the Yentl syndrome, 66-67
Wounds, 185

Yellow/orange vegetables, 147
Yentl syndrome, 66-67
Yogurt, 155-156
Your Body's Many Cries for Water, 215

Zinc, 88, 191-192
Zir, Leonard, 46

Dear Reader:

Thank you for purchasing *Is Heart Surgery Necessary?* by Dr. Julian Whitaker. Regnery Publishing is pleased to bring you high-quality, informative books on preventive medicine. We are dedicated to helping you lead a longer, healthier, and happier life.

If you would like to know more about our books on health-related issues or our classic line of books challenging the status quo, please fill out this postcard and drop it in the mail. Thank you.

Sincerely,

Alfred S. Regnery

Alfred S. Regnery
Publisher

REGNERY PUBLISHING, INC.
Established 1947

Name ❑ Mr. ❑ Mrs. ❑ Miss ❑ Ms. _____

Address _____

City _____ State _____ Zip _____

I would be interested in seeing a book about _____

Health & Healing newsletter order form

Yes! **I agree with Dr. Julian Whitaker** and would like to start on the journey toward creating better health. Please enter my charter subscription, for the term indicated below, and send me Dr. Whitaker's special report, *129 Amazing Medical Secrets*, FREE!

❑ Please sign me up for a one-year subscription to *Health & Healing* for only $39.95. Also send me *129 Amazing Medical Secrets*, Free.

❑ Please sign me up for a two-year subscription for only $79.90. Please include my free copy of Dr. Whitaker's report, *129 Amazing Medical Secrets*.

Method of payment:

❑ Check or money order enclosed for $_____ (Please make your check payable to *Health & Healing*, Maryland residents, please add 5% sales tax.)

❑ Please charge my: ❑ Visa ❑ MasterCard ❑ Discover

Card # _____ Expires _____

Name _____

Address _____

City _____ State _____ Zip _____

Daytime Phone ( ) _____

Signature _____
(necessary for credit card orders)

Please send this order form and your payment to:

Dr. Julian Whitaker's *Health & Healing* • 7811 Montrose Road, Potomac, MD 20854
For faster Service: **Call toll-free 1-800-777-5005.** (Please have your credit card handy)

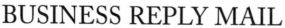

JE/HDN

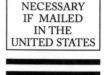

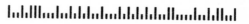